P9-DGL-656

Workbook to Accompany

The
Medical
Manager®
for Windows®

STUDENT EDITION
VERSION 10

Workbook to Accompany

The Medical Manager® for Windows®

STUDENT EDITION
VERSION 10

Computerized Practice Management

Richard Gartee
Medical Manager
Research & Development
Alachua, Florida

Prepared by Maria Citera

THOMSON
─*─
DELMAR LEARNING™   Australia Canada Mexico Singapore Spain United Kingdom United States

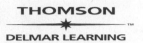

THOMSON

DELMAR LEARNING

Workbook to Accompany The Medical Manager® Student Edition
Version 10 for Windows®

by Richard Gartee

Prepared by Maria Citera

Vice President, Health Care Business Unit:
William Brottmiller

Editorial Director:
Cathy L. Esperti

Acquisitions Editor:
Rhonda Dearborn

Developmental Editor:
Mary Ellen Cox

Marketing Director:
Jennifer McAvey

Marketing Channel Manager:
Lisa Osgood

Marketing Coordinator:
Mona Caron

Editorial Assistant:
Natalie Wager

Art/Design Coordinator:
Connie Lundberg-Watkins

Project Editor:
Daniel Branagh

Production Coordinator:
Jessica Peterson

COPYRIGHT © 2004 by Medical Manager Research & Development, Inc.

Printed in the United States of America
4 5 XXX 07 06 05

For more information, contact Delmar Learning, 5 Maxwell Drive, Clifton Park, NY 12065
Or find us on the World Wide Web at
http://www.delmarlearning.com

ALL RIGHTS RESERVED. No part of this work covered by the copyright hereon may be reproduced or used in any form or by any means—graphic, electronic, or mechanical, including photocopying, recording, taping, Web distribution or information storage and retrieval systems—without the written permission of the publisher.

For permission to use material from this text or product, contact us by
Tel (800) 730-2214
Fax (800) 730-2215
www.thomsonrights.com

ISBN 1-4018-2575-3

Notice to the Reader

Publisher does not warrant or guarantee any of the products described herein or perform any independent analysis in connection with any of the product information contained herein. Publisher does not assume, and expressly disclaims, any obligation to obtain and include information other than that provided to it by the manufacturer.

The reader is expressly warned to consider and adopt all safety precautions that might be indicated by the activities described herein and to avoid all potential hazards. By following the instructions contained herein, the reader willingly assumes all risks in connection with such instructions.

The publisher makes no representations or warranties of any kind, including but not limited to, the warranties of fitness for particular purpose or merchantability, nor are any such representations implied with respect to the material set forth herein, and the publisher takes no responsibility with respect to such material. The publisher shall not be liable for any special, consequential, or exemplary damages resulting, in whole or part, from the reader's use of, or reliance upon, this material.

The Medical Manager and ULTIA are registered trademarks of Medical Manager Research & Development, Inc.

Windows is a registered trademark of Microsoft Corporation.

CONTENTS

P R E F A C E

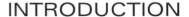

INTRODUCTION

This is a workbook designed to accompany **The Medical Manager** Student Edition, Version 10, for Windows. The purpose for this workbook is to supply the student with additional exercises that coincide with each unit from the Student Edition. By completing these additional exercises, the student can reinforce skills learned and gain confidence by demonstrating the ability to use **The Medical Manager** software.

DEVELOPMENT OF TEXT

This workbook was developed to provide students with supplementary material to complement the coursework from **The Medical Manager** Student Edition, Version 10, for Windows. Many times a student needs additional assignments in order to understand a concept or practice a skill. Other times, a student may want to work on additional assignments in order to gain more experience and knowledge. The idea behind this workbook was to assist all students so that they may become proficient in using **The Medical Manager**. In addition, the instructor may use this workbook for competency exercises, unit tests, or to evaluate a student's progress.

ORGANIZATION

Each unit in the Student Edition focuses on specific tasks. The workbook exercises relate to each unit, providing situations that help to emphasize key points and highlight certain features.

The workbook exercises are designed with a brief explanation of the tasks expected to be completed, specific exercise goals, and relevant questions to consider before entering data. Comprehensive exercises can be found at the end of Unit 8 to help the student feel self-assured as well as allow the instructor to evaluate a student's understanding of **The Medical Manager**.

FEATURES

All exercises are clearly identified in the Contents for easy access. If a student is struggling with a particular task or wants to complete additional work, the Contents can be used to locate exercises utilizing the designed function.

A student data disk has been provided with the workbook. This data disk contains the data necessary to complete the unit exercises.

In addition to the exercises, images of **The Medical Manager** screens are provided in order to check data entered. By using the screen images, a student can identify any errors in entry and/or ensure the accuracy of each posting.

HOW TO USE

A student can easily use this workbook to enhance the skills learned from the Student Edition. For best benefits, after completing each unit from **The Medical Manager** Student Edition, Version 10, for Windows, it is suggested that students follow through all the unit exercises provided in the workbook. In this way, a student will gain optimal experience at using this software.

If it is not possible to complete all the additional exercises from the workbook, a student or instructor may select particular exercises to review. Each unit in the workbook is independent of the other. For example, a student need not complete the exercises from Unit 3 before attempting exercises from Unit 4. The student data disk contains the information necessary for each task.

Instructors may choose to use this workbook for unit tests. Each exercise is given a brief explanation or goal of the task at hand; however, step-by-step instructions are not provided. In this way, a student will need to retain and recall information provided from the Student Edition exercises.

Whatever the needs of the individual student or entire class, **The Medical Manager** Student Edition Workbook provides the tools necessary to be a successful user of **The Medical Manager** software program.

ABOUT THE AUTHORS

Richard Gartee is Director of Design Strategy at Medical Manager Research & Development, Inc., the company that authors **The Medical Manager** software. He serves as part of **The Medical Manager** program design team. He also developed the original dealer and end-user training programs under which more than 200 dealerships and 24,000 medical offices have been trained.

Richard Gartee is one of the original coauthors, and editor of **The Medical Manager** documentation, as well as numerous specialized training guides. He designs new modules of **The Medical Manager** software. He serves as Medical Manager Research & Development, Inc.'s liaison to IBM, Blue Cross/Blue Shield, and other companies in the computer industry as well as the U.S. Department of Commerce International Trade Administration and various universities. He is listed in Who's Who in America and Who's Who in the Computer Industry.

Maria Citera is a professor at Briarcliffe College, New York. Prior to teaching, she had worked in pediatrics for nine years as a medical receptionist, medical biller, and medical assistant. Later she worked at a clinic as an office manager, as well as provided training at various sites on **The Medical Manager** software. She has grown with **The Medical Manager** from the DOS version to version 10.

Maria Citera has been an educator for the past eight years, with a specialty in the medical field. Among various computer courses, she teaches medical terminology, medical transcription, medical coding and insurance procedures, and **The Medical Manager** software program to students preparing to enter the medical office profession.

Using The
Medical Manager

EXERCISE 1: REGISTER YOUR STUDENT NAME

If you are not already logged into **The Medical Manager**, insert the student disk from the workbook and do so at this time.

Type /C2 and press ENTER.
Choose option 11, Student Name Registration.
Enter your first and last name and press PROCESS.
Exit and re-enter **The Medical Manager**.

EXERCISE 2: FLOW OF INFORMATION IN A MEDICAL OFFICE

Answer the following questions based on your understanding and review of Unit 1.

1. Discuss the importance of the flow of information in a medical office.

_____

_____

_____

_____

_____

2. Define overbooking and describe why it is not recommended.

_____

_____

_____

_____

_____

3. Name three situations that you would consider an emergency for a patient.

1. _____

2. _____

3. _____

4. What information is found on an encounter form?

_____

_____

5. Describe the main goal of managed care plans.

_____

_____

_____

6. What does 'PCP' stand for?

_____

7. Name five practice management advantages of **The Medical Manager** software.

　　1. _____

　　2. _____

　　3. _____

　　4. _____

　　5. _____

8. Describe how the mouse and keyboard can be used for direct chaining.

_____

_____

_____

_____

9. What edit key will erase all characters in the field?

_____

10. What key is used to process data and save your work?

_____

11. Discuss the importance of the File Maintenance menu.

_____

_____

_____

_____

12. What key is the same as keying a '?' to open help windows?

_____

13. A CPT-4 code is what type of medical code?

_____

14. An ICD-9 code is what type of medical code?

15. What does a fatal error indicate?

_____

_____

_____

U N I T 2

Building Your Patient File

In the unit exercises that follow (Accounts 300–304) you will be entering new patient accounts from the patient registration forms provided.

EXERCISE 1: PATIENT WITH GUARANTOR INSURANCE

THERESA WALTERS; ACCOUNT 300

1. Before attempting data entry, study the patient registration form in Figure 2-1 (page 4). Answer the following questions:

   a. Who is the guarantor for the account? _____

   b. What is the relationship between the guarantor and the patient? _____

   c. Is Extended Information provided for Theresa Walters? _____

   d. How many insurance policies are there for the account? _____

   e. Who is the policyholder of the insurance? _____

Figure 2-1 Patient Registration – Theresa Walters

Patient Registration Form

Sydney Carrington & Associates
34 Sycamore Street ● Madison, CA 95653

<table>
<tr><td colspan="2"></td><td>

FOR OFFICE USE ONLY

</td></tr>
<tr><td>TODAY'S DATE: _04/16/2003_</td><td></td><td>

ACCOUNT NO.:	**300**
DOCTOR:	**#1**
BILL TYPE:	**11**
EXTENDED INFO.:	**2**

</td></tr>
</table>

PATIENT INFORMATION	GUARANTOR INFORMATION

PATIENT INFORMATION

Walters	Theresa		L.
PATIENT LAST NAME	FIRST NAME		MI

Wife
RELATIONSHIP TO GUARANTOR

F	05/10/1974	Married	132-17-0427
SEX (M/F)	DATE OF BIRTH	MARITAL STATUS	SOC. SEC. #

EMPLOYER OR SCHOOL NAME

ADDRESS OF EMPLOYER OR SCHOOL

CITY	STATE	ZIP CODE

Katrina Johnson, M.D.

EMPLOYER OR SCHOOL PHONE	REFERRED BY

E-MAIL

GUARANTOR INFORMATION

Walters	Charles	–	M
RESPONSIBLE PARTY LAST NAME	FIRST NAME	MI	SEX (M/F)

3 Jefferson Avenue

MAILING ADDRESS	STREET ADDRESS (IF DIFFERENT)

Floral City		CA	94064
CITY		STATE	ZIP CODE

(916) 752-9612	(917) 529-7788
(AREA CODE) HOME PHONE	(AREA CODE) WORK PHONE

03/19/1970	Married	145-98-0424
DATE OF BIRTH	MARITAL STATUS	SOC. SEC. #

Otis Electronics
EMPLOYER NAME

18 Saxon Avenue
EMPLOYER ADDRESS

Madison		CA	95653
CITY		STATE	ZIP CODE

PRIMARY INSURANCE	SECONDARY INSURANCE

PRIMARY INSURANCE

Cross and Shield Ins.
NAME OF PRIMARY INSURANCE COMPANY

435 Embarcadero
ADDRESS

Madison		CA	95653
CITY		STATE	ZIP CODE

145980424	Otis	
IDENTIFICATION #		GROUP NAME AND/OR #

Charles Walters
INSURED PERSON'S NAME (IF DIFFERENT FROM THE RESPONSIBLE PARTY)

Same
ADDRESS (IF DIFFERENT)

Same		
CITY	STATE	ZIP CODE

(800) 345-7689	145-98-0424
PRIMARY INSURANCE PHONE NUMBER	SOC. SEC. #

Self
WHAT IS THE RESPONSIBLE PARTY'S RELATIONSHIP TO THE INSURED?

SECONDARY INSURANCE

NAME OF SECONDARY INSURANCE COMPANY

ADDRESS

CITY	STATE	ZIP CODE

IDENTIFICATION #	GROUP NAME AND/OR #

INSURED PERSON'S NAME (IF DIFFERENT FROM THE RESPONSIBLE PARTY)

ADDRESS (IF DIFFERENT)

CITY	STATE	ZIP CODE

SECONDARY INSURANCE PHONE NUMBER	SOC. SEC. #

WHAT IS THE RESPONSIBLE PARTY'S RELATIONSHIP TO THE INSURED?

I hereby consent for Sydney Carrington & Associates, P.A. to use or disclose my health information to carry out treatment, payment, and health care operations. I authorize the use of this signature on all insurance submissions. I understand that I am financially responsible for all charges whether or not paid by the insurance. I acknowledge receipt of the practice's privacy policy.

Theresa L. Walters	_04/16/2003_
PATIENT SIGNATURE	DATE

2. Based on the information found on the patient registration form, add Theresa Walters as a new patient. Compare your screens to Figures 2-2 through 2-6.

Figure 2-2 Guarantor Information

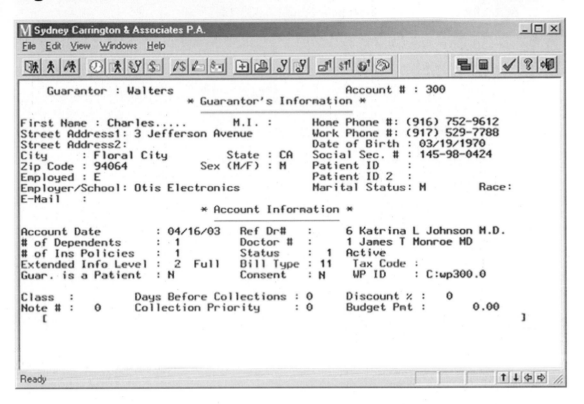

Figure 2-3 Guarantor Extended Information

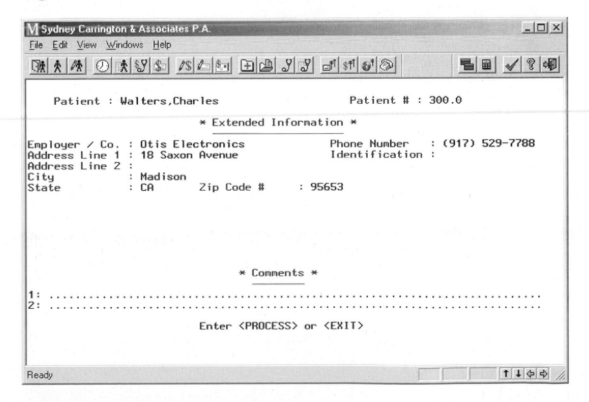

Figure 2-4 Theresa Walters Information

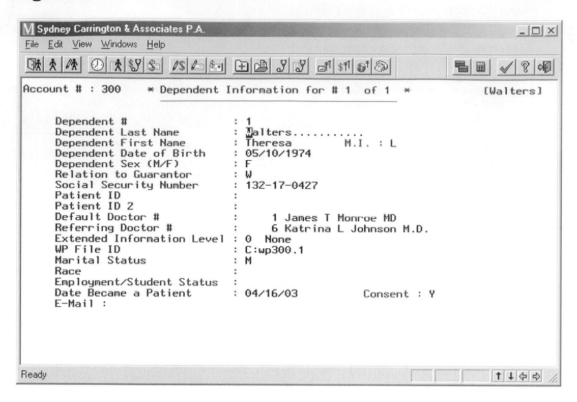

```
M Sydney Carrington & Associates P.A.                              _ □ ×
 File  Edit  View  Windows  Help

 [toolbar icons]                                    [toolbar icons]

 Account # : 300      * Dependent Information for # 1  of 1  *        [Walters]
                      _____

          Dependent #                 : 1
          Dependent Last Name         : Walters...........
          Dependent First Name        : Theresa        M.I. : L
          Dependent Date of Birth     : 05/10/1974
          Dependent Sex (M/F)         : F
          Relation to Guarantor       : W
          Social Security Number      : 132-17-0427
          Patient ID                  :
          Patient ID 2                :
          Default Doctor #            :      1 James T Monroe MD
          Referring Doctor #          :      6 Katrina L Johnson M.D.
          Extended Information Level  : 0  None
          WP File ID                  : C:wp300.1
          Marital Status              : M
          Race                        :
          Employment/Student Status   :
          Date Became a Patient       : 04/16/03        Consent : Y
          E-Mail :

 Ready                                                        ↑ ↓ ⇦ ⇨
```

Figure 2-5 Insurance Policy – Walters

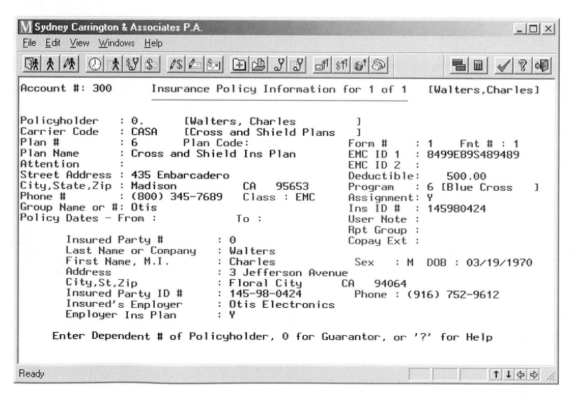

```
M Sydney Carrington & Associates P.A.                              _ □ ×
 File  Edit  View  Windows  Help

 [toolbar icons]                                    [toolbar icons]

 Account #: 300        Insurance Policy Information for 1 of 1   [Walters,Charles]
                       _____

 Policyholder    : 0.      [Walters, Charles        ]
 Carrier Code    : CASA    [Cross and Shield Plans   ]
 Plan #          : 6       Plan Code:             Form #    : 1   Fmt # : 1
 Plan Name       : Cross and Shield Ins Plan     EMC ID 1  : 8499E89S489489
 Attention       :                               EMC ID 2  :
 Street Address  : 435 Embarcadero               Deductible:    500.00
 City,State,Zip  : Madison       CA    95653     Program   : 6 [Blue Cross    ]
 Phone #         : (800) 345-7689   Class : EMC  Assignment: Y
 Group Name or #: Otis                           Ins ID #  : 145980424
 Policy Dates - From :            To :           User Note :
                                                 Rpt Group :
           Insured Party #       : 0            Copay Ext :
           Last Name or Company  : Walters
           First Name, M.I.      : Charles        Sex  : M  DOB : 03/19/1970
           Address               : 3 Jefferson Avenue
           City,St,Zip           : Floral City    CA    94064
           Insured Party ID #    : 145-98-0424   Phone : (916) 752-9612
           Insured's Employer    : Otis Electronics
           Employer Ins Plan     : Y

      Enter Dependent # of Policyholder, 0 for Guarantor, or '?' for Help

 Ready                                                        ↑ ↓ ⇦ ⇨
```

Figure 2-6 Insurance Coverage – Walters

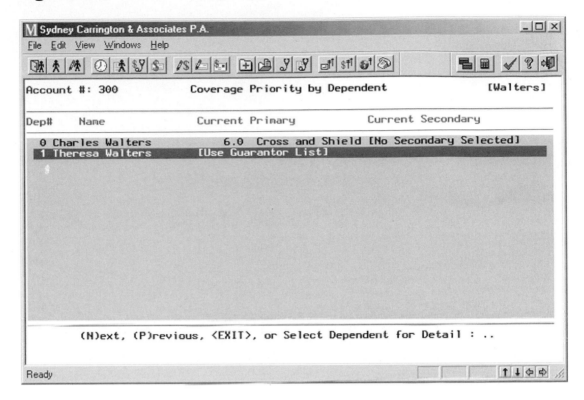

EXERCISE 2: PATIENT WITH DIFFERENT LAST NAME AND DIFFERENT INSURED PARTY

HELENA CARLOS; ACCOUNT 301

1. Before attempting data entry, study the patient registration form in Figure 2-7. Answer the following questions.

    a. What is the relationship between the guarantor, patient, and policyholder? _____

    b. In the Employed field, will Helena be (E)mployed, (P)art Time Student, or (F)ull Time Student? _____

    c. What is the address of the policyholder? _____

       Is it different from the guarantor's address? _____

Figure 2-7 Patient Registration – Helena Carlos

FOR OFFICE USE ONLY	
ACCOUNT NO.:	301
DOCTOR:	#1
BILL TYPE:	11
EXTENDED INFO.:	0

Patient Registration Form

Sydney Carrington & Associates
34 Sycamore Street ● Madison, CA 95653

TODAY'S DATE: _04/16/2003_

PATIENT INFORMATION

Carlos	Helena	
PATIENT LAST NAME	FIRST NAME	MI
Daughter		
RELATIONSHIP TO GUARANTOR		
F	01/19/1987	Single	413-02-5630
SEX (M/F)	DATE OF BIRTH	MARITAL STATUS	SOC. SEC. #
Floral City High School		
EMPLOYER OR SCHOOL NAME		

ADDRESS OF EMPLOYER OR SCHOOL

Floral City	CA	94064
CITY	STATE	ZIP CODE

EMPLOYER OR SCHOOL PHONE   REFERRED BY

E-MAIL

GUARANTOR INFORMATION

Rojas	Yvonne	M	F
RESPONSIBLE PARTY LAST NAME	FIRST NAME	MI	SEX (M/F)
11 Rumpford Avenue			
MAILING ADDRESS		STREET ADDRESS (IF DIFFERENT)	
Floral City	CA	94064
CITY	STATE	ZIP CODE
(916) 818-2461		
(AREA CODE) HOME PHONE		(AREA CODE) WORK PHONE
05/30/1960	Married	192-83-7662
DATE OF BIRTH	MARITAL STATUS	SOC. SEC. #

EMPLOYER NAME

EMPLOYER ADDRESS

	STATE	ZIP CODE
CITY		

PRIMARY INSURANCE

Epsilon Life & Casualty
NAME OF PRIMARY INSURANCE COMPANY

P.O. Box 189
ADDRESS

Macon	GA	31298
CITY	STATE	ZIP CODE

067152316	Randall, Inc.
IDENTIFICATION #	GROUP NAME AND/OR #

Luis Carlos
INSURED PERSON'S NAME (IF DIFFERENT FROM THE RESPONSIBLE PARTY)

40 Barker Street
ADDRESS (IF DIFFERENT)

Madison	CA	95653-0235
CITY	STATE	ZIP CODE

(800) 908-7654	067-15-2316
PRIMARY INSURANCE PHONE NUMBER	SOC. SEC. #

Ex-wife
WHAT IS THE RESPONSIBLE PARTY'S RELATIONSHIP TO THE INSURED?

SECONDARY INSURANCE

NAME OF SECONDARY INSURANCE COMPANY

ADDRESS

	STATE	ZIP CODE
CITY		

IDENTIFICATION #	GROUP NAME AND/OR #

INSURED PERSON'S NAME (IF DIFFERENT FROM THE RESPONSIBLE PARTY)

ADDRESS (IF DIFFERENT)

	STATE	ZIP CODE
CITY		

SECONDARY INSURANCE PHONE NUMBER	SOC. SEC. #

WHAT IS THE RESPONSIBLE PARTY'S RELATIONSHIP TO THE INSURED?

I hereby consent for Sydney Carrington & Associates, P.A. to use or disclose my health information to carry out treatment, payment, and health care operations. I authorize the use of this signature on all insurance submissions. I understand that I am financially responsible for all charges whether or not paid by the insurance. I acknowledge receipt of the practice's privacy policy.

Yvonne M. Rojas (Mother)	_04/16/2003_
PATIENT SIGNATURE	DATE

2. Based on the information found on the patient registration form, add Helena Carlos as a new patient. Compare your screens to Figures 2-8 through 2-12.

Figure 2-8 Guarantor Information – Rojas

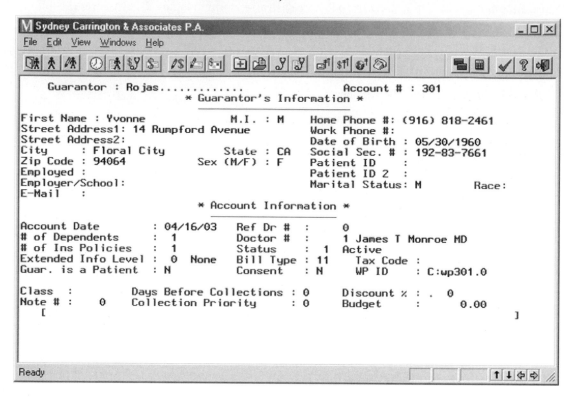

Figure 2-9 Dependent Information – Carlos

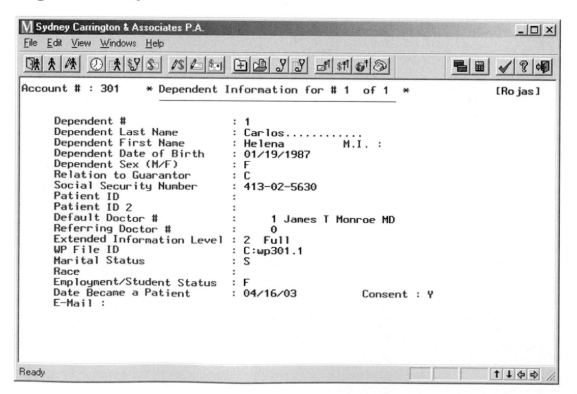

UNIT 2 Building Your Patient File

Figure 2-10 Extended Information – Carlos

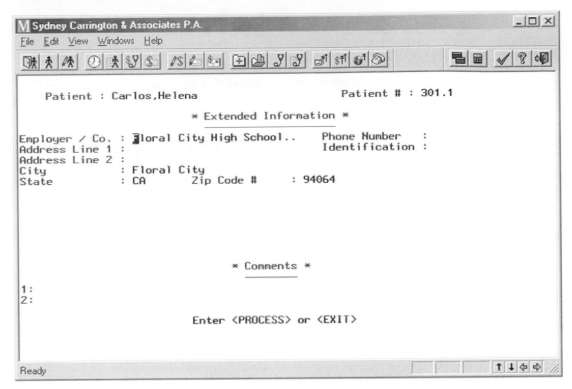

NOTE: *Insured party numbers are assigned by the computer and may differ from the number shown in Figure 2-11.*

Figure 2-11 Insurance Policy Information – Carlos

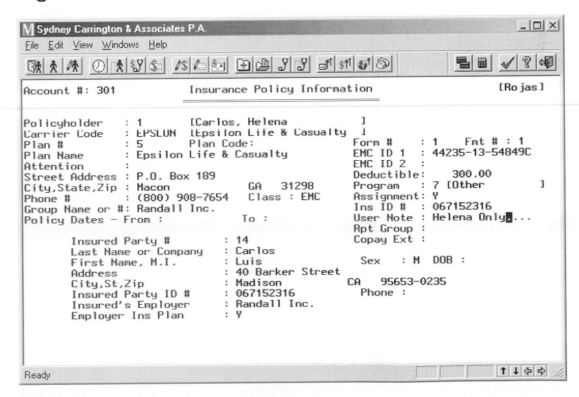

Figure 2-12 Insurance Coverage – Carlos

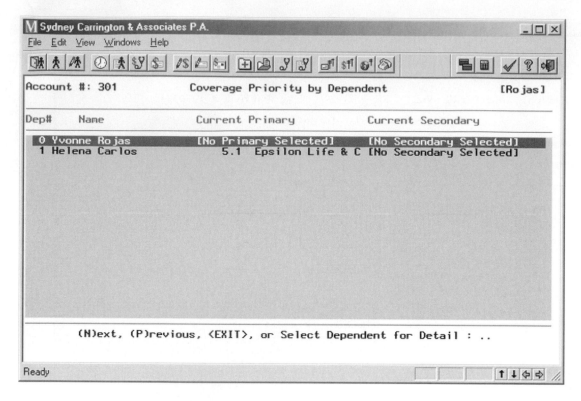

UNIT 2 Building Your Patient File

EDWARD GLENMORE; ACCOUNT 302

1. Before attempting data entry, study the patient registration form in Figure 2-13. Answer the following questions.

   a. What is the address of the patient? _____

      What will appear on Address Line 1? _____

      What will appear on Address Line 2? _____

   b. Who is the policyholder of the insurance? _____

Figure 2-13 Patient Registration – Edward Glenmore

Patient Registration Form

Sydney Carrington & Associates
34 Sycamore Street ● Madison, CA 95653

TODAY'S DATE: _04/16/2003_

FOR OFFICE USE ONLY	
ACCOUNT NO.:	302
DOCTOR:	#2
BILL TYPE:	11
EXTENDED INFO.:	2

PATIENT INFORMATION

Glenmore	Edward	R.
PATIENT LAST NAME	FIRST NAME	MI
Self		
RELATIONSHIP TO GUARANTOR		
M	08/16/1950	Married	147-53-1990
SEX (M/F)	DATE OF BIRTH	MARITAL STATUS	SOC. SEC. #
Powers Lighting, Inc.		
EMPLOYER OR SCHOOL NAME		
P.O. Box 426		
ADDRESS OF EMPLOYER OR SCHOOL		
Madison	CA	95653-0235
CITY	STATE	ZIP CODE
(916) 334-9800		
EMPLOYER OR SCHOOL PHONE	REFERRED BY	
E-MAIL		

GUARANTOR INFORMATION

Glenmore	Edward	R.	M
RESPONSIBLE PARTY LAST NAME	FIRST NAME	MI	SEX (M/F)
P.O. Box 1624	12 Kenway Street		
MAILING ADDRESS	STREET ADDRESS (IF DIFFERENT)		
Madison	CA	95653-0235	
CITY	STATE	ZIP CODE	
(916) 707-1531	(916) 334-9800		
(AREA CODE) HOME PHONE	(AREA CODE) WORK PHONE		
08/16/1950	Married	147-53-1990	
DATE OF BIRTH	MARITAL STATUS	SOC. SEC. #	
Powers Lighting, Inc.			
EMPLOYER NAME			
P.O. Box 426			
EMPLOYER ADDRESS			
Madison	CA	95653-0235	
CITY	STATE	ZIP CODE	

PRIMARY INSURANCE

Fringe Benefits Center		
NAME OF PRIMARY INSURANCE COMPANY		
123 Mission Corners		
ADDRESS		
San Mateo	TX	78723
CITY	STATE	ZIP CODE
14876PL	Powers	
IDENTIFICATION #	GROUP NAME AND/OR #	
Powers Lighting, Inc.		
INSURED PERSON'S NAME (IF DIFFERENT FROM THE RESPONSIBLE PARTY)		
P.O. Box 426		
ADDRESS (IF DIFFERENT)		
Madison	CA	95653-0235
CITY	STATE	ZIP CODE
(800) 999-1234	192-76-1544	
PRIMARY INSURANCE PHONE NUMBER	SOC. SEC. #	
Other		
WHAT IS THE RESPONSIBLE PARTY'S RELATIONSHIP TO THE INSURED?		

SECONDARY INSURANCE

NAME OF SECONDARY INSURANCE COMPANY		
ADDRESS		
CITY	STATE	ZIP CODE
IDENTIFICATION #	GROUP NAME AND/OR #	
INSURED PERSON'S NAME (IF DIFFERENT FROM THE RESPONSIBLE PARTY)		
ADDRESS (IF DIFFERENT)		
CITY	STATE	ZIP CODE
SECONDARY INSURANCE PHONE NUMBER	SOC. SEC. #	
WHAT IS THE RESPONSIBLE PARTY'S RELATIONSHIP TO THE INSURED?		

I hereby consent for Sydney Carrington & Associates, P.A. to use or disclose my health information to carry out treatment, payment, and health care operations. I authorize the use of this signature on all insurance submissions. I understand that I am financially responsible for all charges whether or not paid by the insurance. I acknowledge receipt of the practice's privacy policy.

Edward R. Glenmore   04/16/2003
PATIENT SIGNATURE   DATE

---

2. Based on the information found on the patient registration form, add Edward Glenmore as a new patient. Compare your screens to Figures 2-14 through 2-17.

Figure 2-14 Guarantor Information – Glenmore

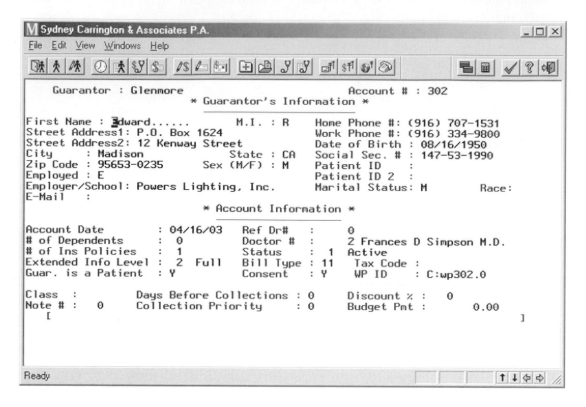

Figure 2-15 Guarantor Extended Information – Glenmore

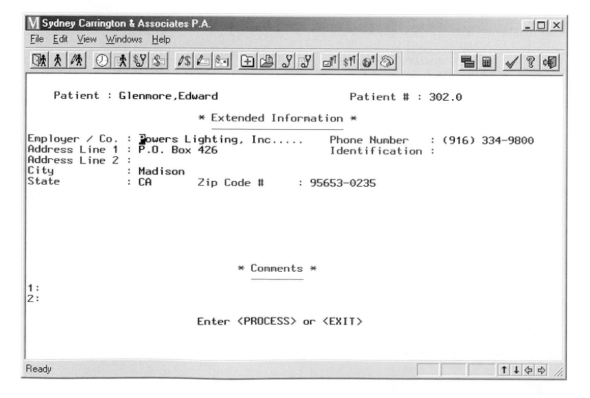

Figure 2-16 Insurance Policy – Glenmore

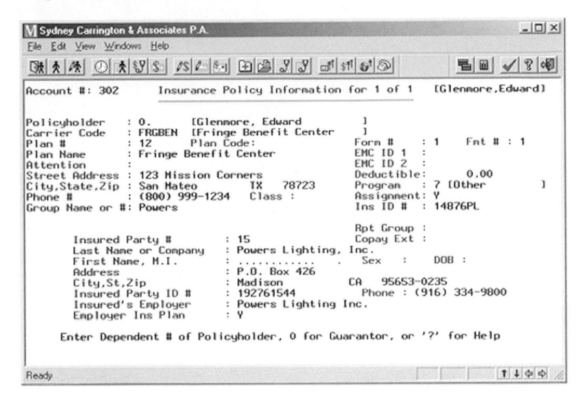

Figure 2-17 Insurance Coverage – Glenmore

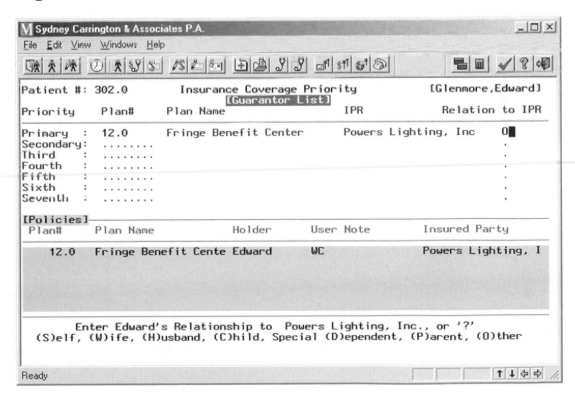

EXERCISE 4: MULTIPLE INSURANCE PLANS

NANCY MONACO; ACCOUNT 303

1. Before attempting data entry, study the patient registration form in Figure 2-18. Answer the following questions.

   a. How many insurances are there? _____

   b. Who is the policyholder of the primary insurance? _____

      Who is the policyholder of the secondary insurance?_____

   c. What is the relationship between the guarantor and the patient?_____

Figure 2-18 Patient Registration – Nancy Monaco

Patient Registration Form

Sydney Carrington & Associates
34 Sycamore Street ● Madison, CA 95653

TODAY'S DATE: _04/16/2003_

FOR OFFICE USE ONLY

ACCOUNT NO.:	**303**
DOCTOR:	**#3**
BILL TYPE:	**11**
EXTENDED INFO.:	**2**

PATIENT INFORMATION

Monaco	_Nancy_	–
PATIENT LAST NAME	FIRST NAME	MI

Wife
RELATIONSHIP TO GUARANTOR

_F_	_07/20/1960_	_Married_	_541-03-1116_
SEX (M/F)	DATE OF BIRTH	MARITAL STATUS	SOC. SEC. #

Alpha Learning Center
EMPLOYER OR SCHOOL NAME

1050 Harper Court
ADDRESS OF EMPLOYER OR SCHOOL

Woodside	_CA_	_98076_
CITY	STATE	ZIP CODE

_(408) 696-2312_	_Richard Bardsley, MD_
EMPLOYER OR SCHOOL PHONE	REFERRED BY

E-MAIL

GUARANTOR INFORMATION

Monaco	_Anthony_	_J._	_M_
RESPONSIBLE PARTY LAST NAME	FIRST NAME	MI	SEX (M/F)

55 Fordham Street
MAILING ADDRESS

STREET ADDRESS (IF DIFFERENT)

Woodside	_CA_	_98076_
CITY	STATE	ZIP CODE

_(408) 476-8521_	_(408) 918-2200_
(AREA CODE) HOME PHONE	(AREA CODE) WORK PHONE

_01/05/1959_	_Married_	_721-44-0809_
DATE OF BIRTH	MARITAL STATUS	SOC. SEC. #

Joe's Auto Body
EMPLOYER NAME

2512 Broadway Avenue
EMPLOYER ADDRESS

Woodside	_CA_	_98076_
CITY	STATE	ZIP CODE

PRIMARY INSURANCE

Epsilon Life & Casualty
NAME OF PRIMARY INSURANCE COMPANY

P.O. Box 189
ADDRESS

Macon	_GA_	_31298_
CITY	STATE	ZIP CODE

_721440809A_	_1298_
IDENTIFICATION #	GROUP NAME AND/OR #

Anthony Monaco
INSURED PERSON'S NAME (IF DIFFERENT FROM THE RESPONSIBLE PARTY)

Same
ADDRESS (IF DIFFERENT)

Same		
CITY	STATE	ZIP CODE

_(800) 908-7654_	_721-44-0809_
PRIMARY INSURANCE PHONE NUMBER	SOC. SEC. #

Self
WHAT IS THE RESPONSIBLE PARTY'S RELATIONSHIP TO THE INSURED?

SECONDARY INSURANCE

Pan American Health Ins.
NAME OF SECONDARY INSURANCE COMPANY

4567 Newberry Road
ADDRESS

Los Angeles	_CA_	_98706_
CITY	STATE	ZIP CODE

_541031116_	_Alpha_
IDENTIFICATION #	GROUP NAME AND/OR #

Nancy Monaco
INSURED PERSON'S NAME (IF DIFFERENT FROM THE RESPONSIBLE PARTY)

Same
ADDRESS (IF DIFFERENT)

Same		
CITY	STATE	ZIP CODE

_(213) 456-7654_	_541-03-1116_
SECONDARY INSURANCE PHONE NUMBER	SOC. SEC. #

Husband
WHAT IS THE RESPONSIBLE PARTY'S RELATIONSHIP TO THE INSURED?

I hereby consent for Sydney Carrington & Associates, P.A. to use or disclose my health information to carry out treatment, payment, and health care operations. I authorize the use of this signature on all insurance submissions. I understand that I am financially responsible for all charges whether or not paid by the insurance. I acknowledge receipt of the practice's privacy policy.

Nancy Monaco	_04/16/2003_
PATIENT SIGNATURE	DATE

2. Based on the information found on the patient registration form, add Nancy Monaco as a new patient. Compare your screens to those shown in Figures 2-19 through 2-25.

Figure 2-19 Guarantor Information – Monaco

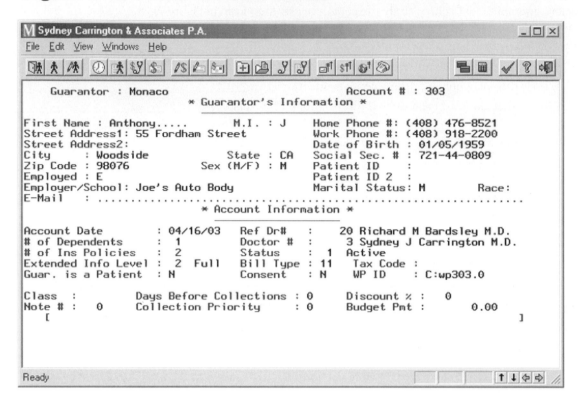

Figure 2-20 Guarantor Extended Information – Monaco

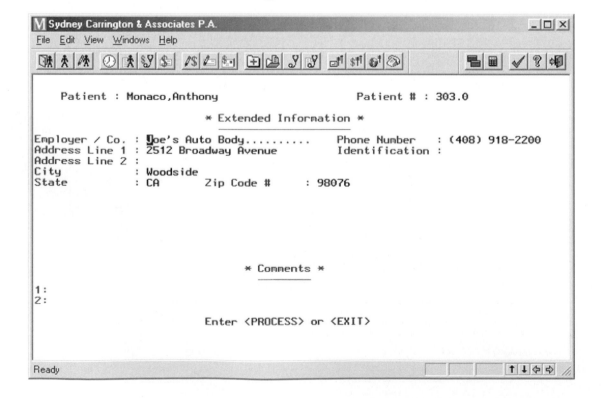

Figure 2-21 Dependent Information – Monaco

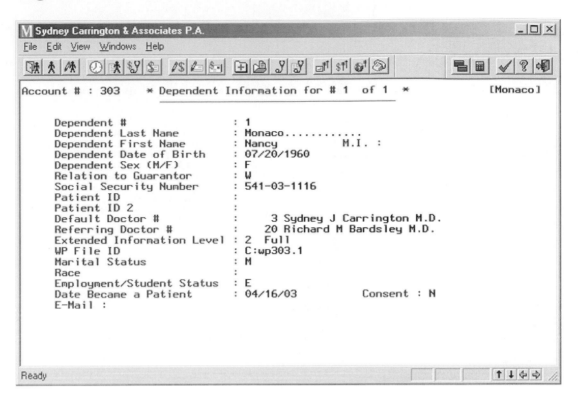

Figure 2-22 Dependent Extended Information – Monaco

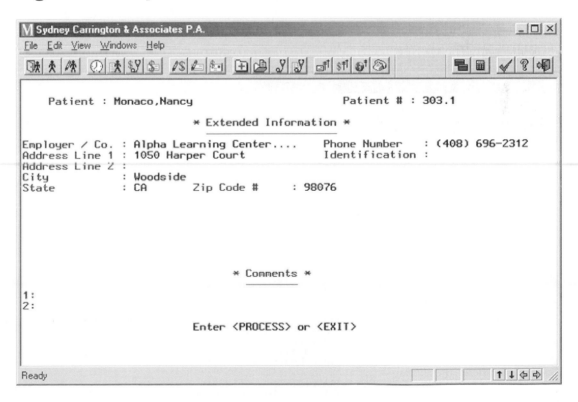

Figure 2-23 Insurance Policy 1 – Monaco

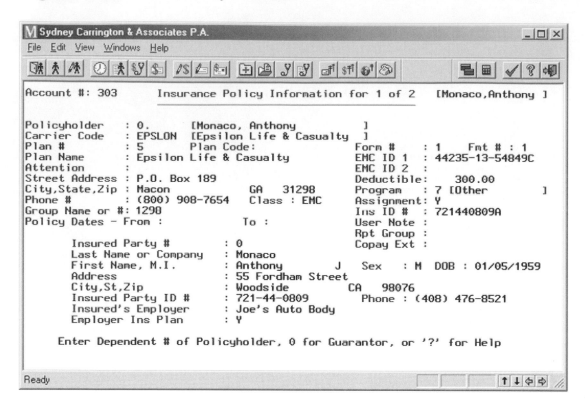

NOTE: *Insured party numbers are assigned by the computer. The insured party number on your screen may differ from that shown in Figure 2-24.*

Figure 2-24 Insurance Policy 2 – Monaco

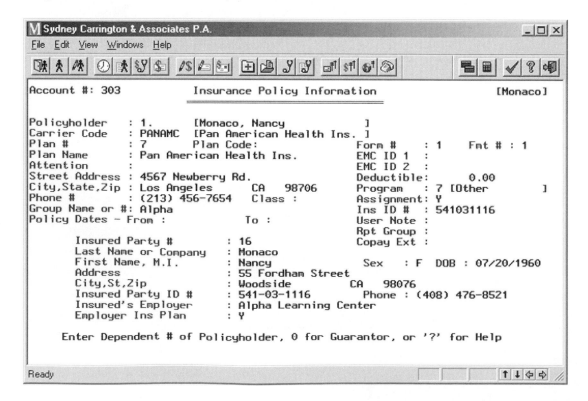

Figure 2-25 Insurance Coverage – Monaco

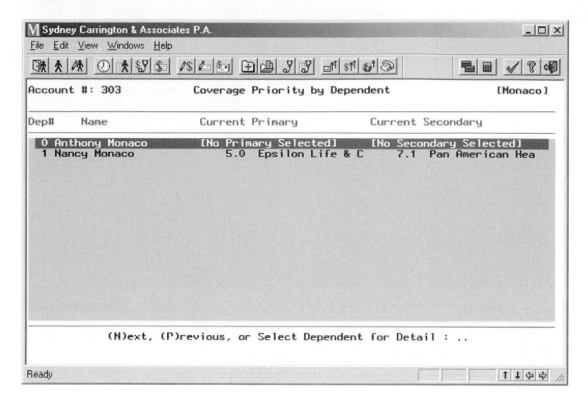

EXERCISE 5: MULTIPLE INSURANCE POLICIES, DIFFERENT INSURED PARTY

VINCENT MONTI; ACCOUNT 304

1. Before attempting data entry, study the patient registration form in Figure 2-26. Answer the following questions.

    a. What is the name of the primary insurance? _____

    b. What is the name of the secondary insurance? _____

    c. Who is the policyholder for each insurance? _____

Figure 2-26 Patient Registration – Vincent Monti

Patient Registration Form

Sydney Carrington & Associates
34 Sycamore Street ● Madison, CA 95653

FOR OFFICE USE ONLY	
ACCOUNT NO.:	304
DOCTOR:	#2
BILL TYPE:	11
EXTENDED INFO.:	2

TODAY'S DATE: _04/16/2003_

PATIENT INFORMATION

Monti	Vincent	A.
PATIENT LAST NAME	FIRST NAME	MI

Self
RELATIONSHIP TO GUARANTOR

M	06/23/1968	Married	116-29-1029
SEX (M/F)	DATE OF BIRTH	MARITAL STATUS	SOC. SEC. #

B.C. Nurseries, Inc.
EMPLOYER OR SCHOOL NAME

136 Concourse Avenue
ADDRESS OF EMPLOYER OR SCHOOL

Wallace	CA	95039
CITY	STATE	ZIP CODE

(916) 971-5381	Leland Groves, MD
EMPLOYER OR SCHOOL PHONE	REFERRED BY

E-MAIL

GUARANTOR INFORMATION

Monti	Vincent	A.	M
RESPONSIBLE PARTY LAST NAME	FIRST NAME	MI	SEX (M/F)

48 Clermont Road
MAILING ADDRESS

Wallace	CA	95039
CITY	STATE	ZIP CODE

(916) 497-5106	(916) 971-5381
(AREA CODE) HOME PHONE	(AREA CODE) WORK PHONE

06/23/1968	Married	116-29-1029
DATE OF BIRTH	MARITAL STATUS	SOC. SEC. #

B.C. Nurseries, Inc.
EMPLOYER NAME

136 Concourse Avenue
EMPLOYER ADDRESS

Wallace	CA	95039
CITY	STATE	ZIP CODE

PRIMARY INSURANCE

Pan American Health Ins.
NAME OF PRIMARY INSURANCE COMPANY

4567 Newberry Road
ADDRESS

Los Angeles	CA	98706
CITY	STATE	ZIP CODE

012440112	
IDENTIFICATION #	GROUP NAME AND/OR #

Sandra B. Monti
INSURED PERSON'S NAME (IF DIFFERENT FROM THE RESPONSIBLE PARTY)

Same
ADDRESS (IF DIFFERENT)

Same		
CITY	STATE	ZIP CODE

(213) 456-7654	012-44-0112
PRIMARY INSURANCE PHONE NUMBER	SOC. SEC. #

Husband
WHAT IS THE RESPONSIBLE PARTY'S RELATIONSHIP TO THE INSURED?

SECONDARY INSURANCE

Epsilon Life & Casualty
NAME OF SECONDARY INSURANCE COMPANY

P.O. Box 189
ADDRESS

Macon	GA	31298
CITY	STATE	ZIP CODE

116291029	BCN
IDENTIFICATION #	GROUP NAME AND/OR #

Vincent A. Monti
INSURED PERSON'S NAME (IF DIFFERENT FROM THE RESPONSIBLE PARTY)

Same
ADDRESS (IF DIFFERENT)

Same		
CITY	STATE	ZIP CODE

(800) 908-7654	116-29-1029
SECONDARY INSURANCE PHONE NUMBER	SOC. SEC. #

Self
WHAT IS THE RESPONSIBLE PARTY'S RELATIONSHIP TO THE INSURED?

I hereby consent for Sydney Carrington & Associates, P.A. to use or disclose my health information to carry out treatment, payment, and health care operations. I authorize the use of this signature on all insurance submissions. I understand that I am financially responsible for all charges whether or not paid by the insurance. I acknowledge receipt of the practice's privacy policy.

Vincent A. Monti	04/16/2003
PATIENT SIGNATURE	DATE

2. Based on the information found on the patient registration form, add Vincent Monti as a new patient. Compare your screens to Figures 2-27 through 2-31.

REMINDER: *If a city does not appear in the HOME menu, press ESCAPE and type the information in the field.*

Figure 2-27 Guarantor Information – Monti

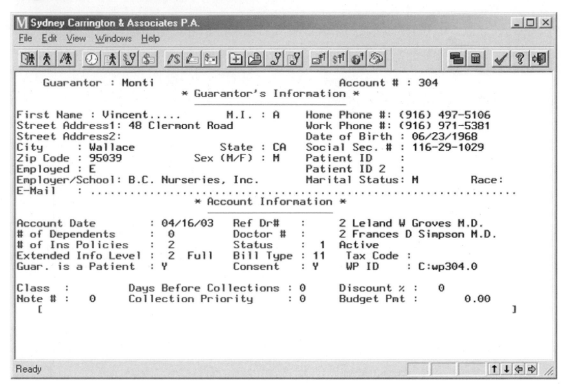

Figure 2-28 Extended Information – Monti

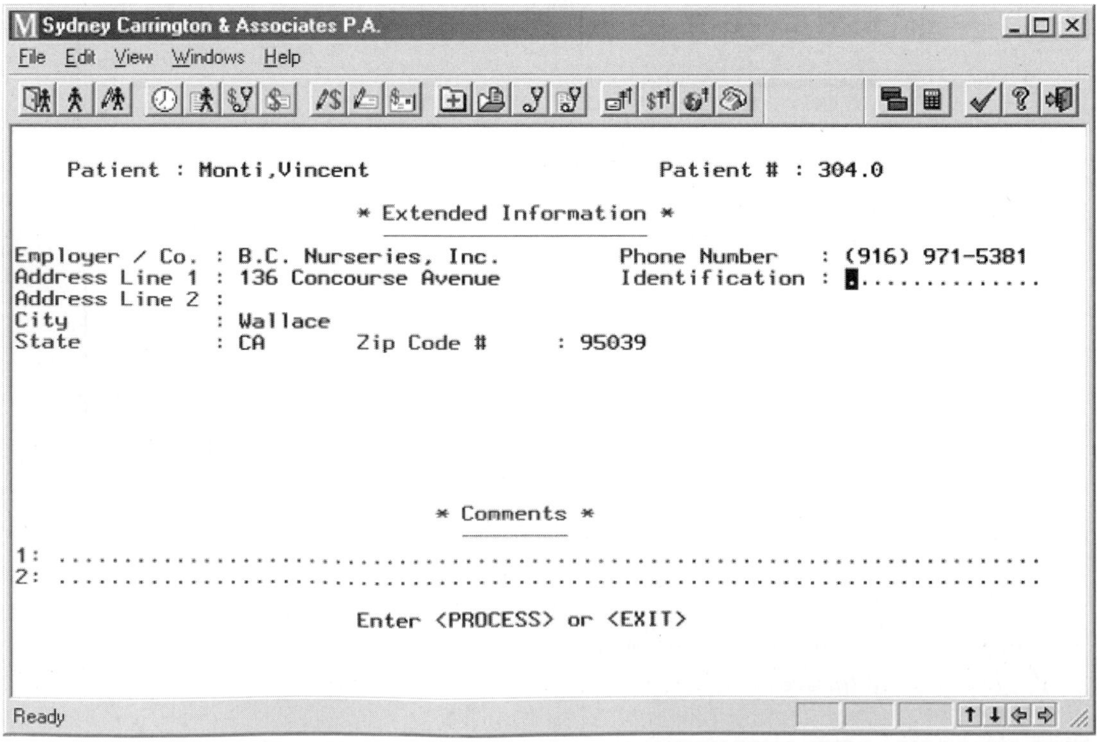

NOTE: Insured party numbers are assigned by the computer. The number assigned in Exercise 5 may differ from that shown in Figure 2-29.

Figure 2-29 Insurance Policy 1 – Monti

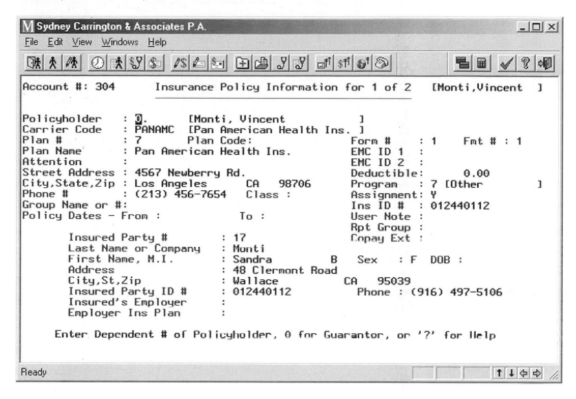

Figure 2-30 Insurance Policy 2 – Monti

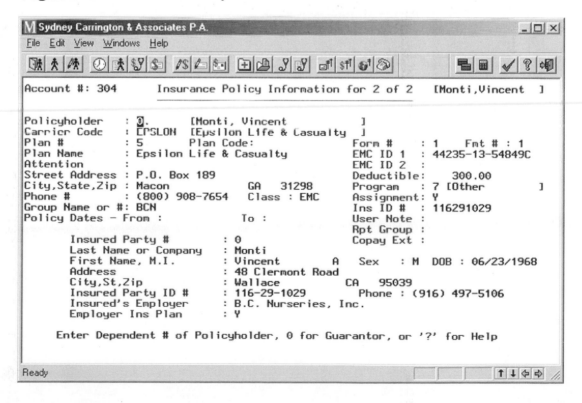

Figure 2-31 Insurance Coverage – Monti

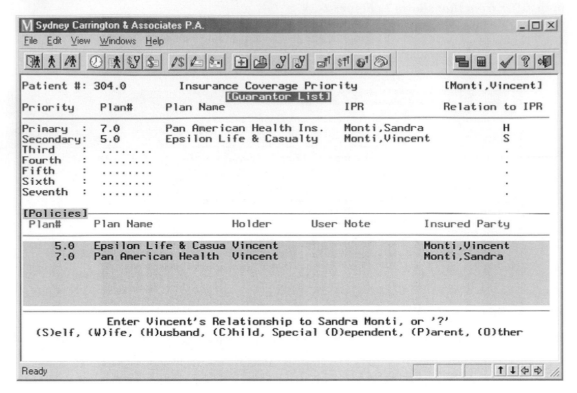

UNIT 2 Building Your Patient File

U N I T 3

Posting Your Entries

In the unit exercises that follow, you will be posting procedure entries from the encounter forms provided.

EXERCISE 1: ONE PROCEDURE, ONE DIAGNOSIS, NO INSURANCE

JUAN PEREZ

GOAL(S): In this exercise you will enter a procedure and diagnosis for a patient with no insurance.

1. Before posting your entry, study the encounter form in Figure 3-1 (page 28). Answer the following questions:

   a. Who is the patient? _____

   b. What is the voucher number on the encounter form? _____

   c. Which doctor saw the patient? _____

   d. How many procedures were completed at this visit? _____

   e. How many diagnoses are listed? _____

Figure 3-1 Encounter Form – Perez

Sydney Carrington & Associates P.A.
34 Sycamore Street   Suite 300
Madison, CA 95653

Date: 04/16/2003   Voucher No.:   4030

Time:

Patient: Juan Perez   Patient No: 309.0
Guarantor: Doctor: 3 - S. Carrington

☐ CPT	DESCRIPTION	FEE	☐ CPT	DESCRIPTION	FEE	☐ CPT	DESCRIPTION	FEE
OFFICE/HOSPITAL CONSULTS			**LABORATORY/RADIOLOGY**			**PROCEDURES/TESTS**		
☐ 99201	Office New:Focused Hx-Exam		☐ 81000	Urinalysis		☐ 00452	Anesthesia for Rad Surgery	
☐ 99202	Office New:Expanded Hx-Exam		☐ 81002	Urinalysis; Pregnancy Test		☐ 11100	Skin Biopsy	
☐ 99211	Office Estb:Min/None Hx-Exa		☐ 82951	Glucose Tolerance Test		☐ 15852	Dressing Change	
☐ 99212	Office Estb:Focused Hx-Exam		☐ 84478	Triglycerides		☐ 29075	Cast Appl. - Lower Arm	
☐ 99213	Office Estb:Expanded Hx-Exa		☐ 84550	Uric Acid: Blood Chemistry		☐ 29530	Strapping of Knee	
☒ 99214	Office Estb:Detailed Hx-Exa		☐ 84830	Ovulation Test		☐ 29705	Removal/Revis of Cast w/Exa	
☐ 99215	Office Estb:Comprhn Hx-Exam		☐ 85014	Hematocrit		☐ 53670	Catheterization Incl. Suppl	
☐ 99221	Hosp. Initial:Comprh Hx-		☐ 85031	Hemogram, Complete Blood Wk		☐ 57452	Colposcopy	
☐ 99223	Hosp.Ini:Comprh Hx-Exam/Hi		☐ 86403	Particle Agglutination Test		☐ 57505	ECC	
☐ 99231	Hosp. Subsequent: S-Fwd		☐ 86485	Skin Test; Candida		☐ 69420	Myringotomy	
☐ 99232	Hosp. Subsequent: Comprhn Hx		☐ 86580	TB Intradermal Test		☐ 92081	Visual Field Examination	
☐ 99233	Hosp. Subsequent: Ex/Hi		☐ 86585	TB Tine Test		☐ 92100	Serial Tonometry Exam	
☐ 99238	Hospital Visit Discharge Ex		☐ 87070	Culture		☐ 92120	Tonography	
☐ 99371	Telephone Consult - Simple		☐ 70190	X-Ray; Optic Foramina		☐ 92552	Pure Tone Audiometry	
☐ 99372	Telephone Consult - Intermed		☐ 70210	X-Ray Sinuses Complete		☐ 92567	Tympanometry	
☐ 99373	Telephone Consult - Complex		☐ 71010	Radiological Exam Ent Spine		☐ 93000	Electrocardiogram	
☐ 90843	Counseling - 25 minutes		☐ 71020	X-Ray Chest Pa & Lat		☐ 93015	Exercise Stress Test (ETT)	
☐ 90844	Counseling - 50 minutes		☐ 72050	X-Ray Spine, Cerv (4 views)		☐ 93017	ETT Tracing Only	
☐ 90865	Counseling - Special Interview		☐ 72090	X-Ray Spine; Scoliosis Ex		☐ 93040	Electrocardiogram - Rhythm	
			☐ 72110	Spine, lumbosacral; a/p & Lat		☐ 96100	Psychological Testing	
IMMUNIZATIONS/INJECTIONS			☐ 73030	Shoulder-Comp, min w/ 2vws		☐ 99000	Specimen Handling	
☐ 90585	BCG Vaccine		☐ 73070	Elbow, anteropost & later vws		☐ 99058	Office Emergency Care	
☐ 90659	Influenza Virus Vaccine		☐ 73120	X-Ray; Hand, 2 views		☐ 99070	Surgical Tray - Misc.	
☐ 90701	Immunization-DTP		☐ 73560	X-Ray, Knee, 1 or 2 views		☐ 99080	Special Reports of Med Rec	
☐ 90702	DT Vaccine		☐ 74022	X-Ray; Abdomen, Complete		☐ 99195	Phlebotomy	
☐ 90703	Tetanus Toxoids		☐ 75552	Cardiac Magnetic Res Img		☐	_____	
☐ 90732	Pneumococcal Vaccine		☐ 76020	X-Ray; Bone Age Studies		☐	_____	
☐ 90746	Hepatitis B Vaccine		☐ 76088	Mammary Ductogram Complete		☐	_____	
☐ 90749	Immunization; Unlisted		☐ 78465	Myocardial Perfusion Img		☐	_____	

ICD-9 CODE DIAGNOSIS		ICD-9 CODE DIAGNOSIS		ICD-9 CODE DIAGNOSIS	
☐ 009.0	Ill-defined Intestinal Infect	☐ 435.0	Basilar Artery Syndrome	☐ 724.2	Pain: Lower Back
☐ 133.2	Establish Baseline	☐ 440.0	Atherosclerosis	☐ 727.6	Rupture of Achilles Tendon
☐ 174.9	Breast Cancer	☐ 442.81	Carotid Artery	☐ 780.1	Hallucinations
☐ 185.0	Prostate Cancer	☐ 460.0	Common Cold	☐ 780.3	Convulsions
☐ 250	Diabetes Mellitus	☐ 461.9	Acute Sinusitis	☐ 780.5	Sleep Disturbances
☐ 272.4	Hyperlipidemia	☐ 474.0	Tonsillitis	☐ 783.0	Anorexia
☐ 282.5	Anemia - Sickle Trait	☐ 477.9	Hay Fever	☐ 783.1	Abnormal Weight Gain
☐ 282.60	Anemia - Sickle Cell	☐ 487.0	Flu	☐ 783.2	Abnormal Weight Loss
☐ 285.9	Anemia, Unspecified	☐ 496	Chronic Airway Obstruction	☐ 830.6	Dislocated Hip
☐ 300.4	Neurotic Depression	☐ 522	Low Red Blood Count	☐ 830.9	Dislocated Shoulder
☐ 340	Multiple Sclerosis	☐ 524.6	Temporo-Mandibular Jnt Synd	☐ 841.2	Sprained Wrist
☐ 342.9	Hemiplegia - Unspecified	☐ 538.8	Stomach Pain	☐ 842.5	Sprained Ankle
☐ 346.9	Migraine Headache	☐ 553.3	Hiatal Hernia	☐ 891.2	Fractured Tibia
☐ 352.9	Cranial Neuralgia	☐ 564.1	Spastic Colon	☐ 892.0	Fractured Fibula
☐ 354.0	Carpal Tunnel Syndrome	☐ 571.4	Chronic Hepatitis	☐ 919.5	Insect Bite, Nonvenomous
☐ 355.0	Sciatic Nerve Root Lesion	☐ 571.5	Cirrhosis of Liver	☐ 921.1	Contus Eyelid/Perioc Area
☐ 366.9	Cataract	☐ 573.3	Hepatitis	☐ v16.3	Fam. Hist of Breast Cancer
☐ 386.0	Vertigo	☐ 575.2	Obstruction of Gallbladder	☐ v17.4	Fam. Hist of Cardiovasc Dis
☒ 401.1	Essential Hypertension	☐ 648.2	Anemia - Compl. Pregnancy	☐ v20.2	Well Child
☐ 414.9	Ischemic Hearth Disease	☐ 715.90	Osteoarthritis - Unspec	☐ v22.0	Pregnancy - First Normal
☐ 428.0	Congestive Heart Failure	☐ 721.3	Lumbar Osteo/Spondylarthrit	☐ v22.1	Pregnancy - Normal

Previous Balance	Today's Charges	Total Due	Amount Paid	New Balance	Follow Up
_____	_____	_____	_____	_____	PRN _____ Weeks _____ Months _____ Units _____

Next Appointment Date: Time:

I hereby authorize release of any information acquired in the course of
examination or treatment and allow a photocopy of my signature to be used.

_____

2. Based on the information found on the encounter form, enter the procedure and diagnosis for Juan Perez. Compare your screen to Figure 3-2.

Figure 3-2 Procedure Entry – Perez

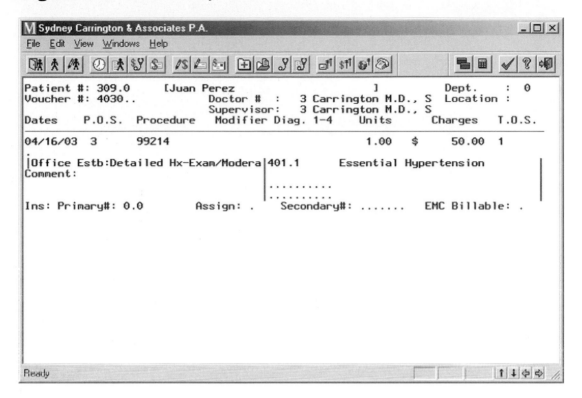

EXERCISE 2: ONE PROCEDURE, ONE DIAGNOSIS, ONE INSURANCE

CATHERINE VIAJO

GOAL(S): In this exercise you will enter a procedure and diagnosis for a patient with one insurance.

1. Before posting your entry, study the encounter form in Figure 3-3 (page 32). Answer the following questions.

   a. Who is the patient? _____

   b. What is the voucher number on the encounter form? _____

   c. Which doctor saw the patient? _____

   d. How many procedures were completed at this visit? _____

   e. How many diagnoses are listed? _____

Figure 3-3 Encounter Form – Viajo

Sydney Carrington & Associates P.A.
34 Sycamore Street   Suite 300
Madison, CA 95653

Date: 04/16/2003

Voucher No.: 4031

Time:

Patient: Catherine Viajo

Patient No: 305.0

Guarantor:

Doctor: 3 - S. Carrington

	CPT	DESCRIPTION	FEE
OFFICE/HOSPITAL CONSULTS			
☐	99201	Office New:Focused Hx-Exam	_____
☐	99202	Office New:Expanded Hx-Exam	_____
☐	99211	Office Estb:Min/None Hx-Exa	_____
☐	99212	Office Estb:Focused Hx-Exam	_____
☒	99213	Office Estb:Expanded Hx-Exa	_____
☐	99214	Office Estb:Detailed Hx-Exa	_____
☐	99215	Office Estb:Comprhn Hx-Exam	_____
☐	99221	Hosp. Initial:Comprh Hx-	_____
☐	99223	Hosp.Ini:Comprh Hx-Exam/Hi	_____
☐	99231	Hosp. Subsequent: S-Fwd	_____
☐	99232	Hosp. Subsequent: Comprhn Hx	_____
☐	99233	Hosp. Subsequent: Ex/Hi	_____
☐	99238	Hospital Visit Discharge Ex	_____
☐	99371	Telephone Consult - Simple	_____
☐	99372	Telephone Consult - Intermed	_____
☐	99373	Telephone Consult - Complex	_____
☐	90843	Counseling - 25 minutes	_____
☐	90844	Counseling - 50 minutes	_____
☐	90865	Counseling - Special Interview	_____
IMMUNIZATIONS/INJECTIONS			
☐	90585	BCG Vaccine	_____
☐	90659	Influenza Virus Vaccine	_____
☐	90701	Immunization-DTP	_____
☐	90702	DT Vaccine	_____
☐	90703	Tetanus Toxoids	_____
☐	90732	Pneumococcal Vaccine	_____
☐	90746	Hepatitis B Vaccine	_____
☐	90749	Immunization; Unlisted	_____

	CPT	DESCRIPTION	FEE
LABORATORY/RADIOLOGY			
☐	81000	Urinalysis	_____
☐	81002	Urinalysis; Pregnancy Test	_____
☐	82951	Glucose Tolerance Test	_____
☐	84478	Triglycerides	_____
☐	84550	Uric Acid: Blood Chemistry	_____
☐	84830	Ovulation Test	_____
☐	85014	Hematocrit	_____
☐	85031	Hemogram, Complete Blood Wk	_____
☐	86403	Particle Agglutination Test	_____
☐	86485	Skin Test; Candida	_____
☐	86580	TB Intradermal Test	_____
☐	86585	TB Tine Test	_____
☐	87070	Culture	_____
☐	70190	X-Ray; Optic Foramina	_____
☐	70210	X-Ray Sinuses Complete	_____
☐	71010	Radiological Exam Ent Spine	_____
☐	71020	X-Ray Chest Pa & Lat	_____
☐	72050	X-Ray Spine, Cerv (4 views)	_____
☐	72090	X-Ray Spine; Scoliosis Ex	_____
☐	72110	Spine, lumbosacral; a/p & Lat	_____
☐	73030	Shoulder-Comp, min w/ 2vws	_____
☐	73070	Elbow, anteropost & later vws	_____
☐	73120	X-Ray; Hand, 2 views	_____
☐	73560	X-Ray, Knee, 1 or 2 views	_____
☐	74022	X-Ray; Abdomen, Complete	_____
☐	75552	Cardiac Magnetic Res Img	_____
☐	76020	X-Ray; Bone Age Studies	_____
☐	76088	Mammary Ductogram Complete	_____
☐	78465	Myocardial Perfusion Img	_____

	CPT	DESCRIPTION	FEE
PROCEDURES/TESTS			
☐	00452	Anesthesia for Rad Surgery	_____
☐	11100	Skin Biopsy	_____
☐	15852	Dressing Change	_____
☐	29075	Cast Appl. - Lower Arm	_____
☐	29530	Strapping of Knee	_____
☐	29705	Removal/Revis of Cast w/Exa	_____
☐	53670	Catheterization Incl. Suppl	_____
☐	57452	Colposcopy	_____
☐	57505	ECC	_____
☐	69420	Myringotomy	_____
☐	92081	Visual Field Examination	_____
☐	92100	Serial Tonometry Exam	_____
☐	92120	Tonography	_____
☐	92552	Pure Tone Audiometry	_____
☐	92567	Tympanometry	_____
☐	93000	Electrocardiogram	_____
☐	93015	Exercise Stress Test (ETT)	_____
☐	93017	ETT Tracing Only	_____
☐	93040	Electrocardiogram - Rhythm	_____
☐	96100	Psychological Testing	_____
☐	99000	Specimen Handling	_____
☐	99058	Office Emergency Care	_____
☐	99070	Surgical Tray - Misc.	_____
☐	99080	Special Reports of Med Rec	_____
☐	99195	Phlebotomy	_____
☐		_____	_____
☐		_____	_____
☐		_____	_____

	ICD-9 CODE DIAGNOSIS	
☐	009.0	Ill-defined Intestinal Infect
☐	133.2	Establish Baseline
☐	174.9	Breast Cancer
☐	185.0	Prostate Cancer
☐	250	Diabetes Mellitus
☐	272.4	Hyperlipidemia
☐	282.5	Anemia - Sickle Trait
☐	282.60	Anemia - Sickle Cell
☐	285.9	Anemia, Unspecified
☐	300.4	Neurotic Depression
☐	340	Multiple Sclerosis
☐	342.9	Hemiplegia - Unspecified
☒	346.9	Migraine Headache
☐	352.9	Cranial Neuralgia
☐	354.0	Carpal Tunnel Syndrome
☐	355.0	Sciatic Nerve Root Lesion
☐	366.9	Cataract
☐	386.0	Vertigo
☐	401.1	Essential Hypertension
☐	414.9	Ischemic Hearth Disease
☐	428.0	Congestive Heart Failure

	ICD-9 CODE DIAGNOSIS	
☐	435.0	Basilar Artery Syndrome
☐	440.0	Atherosclerosis
☐	442.81	Carotid Artery
☐	460.0	Common Cold
☐	461.9	Acute Sinusitis
☐	474.0	Tonsillitis
☐	477.9	Hay Fever
☐	487.0	Flu
☐	496	Chronic Airway Obstruction
☐	522	Low Red Blood Count
☐	524.6	Temporo-Mandibular Jnt Synd
☐	538.8	Stomach Pain
☐	553.3	Hiatal Hernia
☐	564.1	Spastic Colon
☐	571.4	Chronic Hepatitis
☐	571.5	Cirrhosis of Liver
☐	573.3	Hepatitis
☐	575.2	Obstruction of Gallbladder
☐	648.2	Anemia - Compl. Pregnancy
☐	715.90	Osteoarthritis - Unspec
☐	721.3	Lumbar Osteo/Spondylarthrit

	ICD-9 CODE DIAGNOSIS	
☐	724.2	Pain: Lower Back
☐	727.6	Rupture of Achilles Tendon
☐	780.1	Hallucinations
☐	780.3	Convulsions
☐	780.5	Sleep Disturbances
☐	783.0	Anorexia
☐	783.1	Abnormal Weight Gain
☐	783.2	Abnormal Weight Loss
☐	830.6	Dislocated Hip
☐	830.9	Dislocated Shoulder
☐	841.2	Sprained Wrist
☐	842.5	Sprained Ankle
☐	891.2	Fractured Tibia
☐	892.0	Fractured Fibula
☐	919.5	Insect Bite, Nonvenomous
☐	921.1	Contus Eyelid/Perioc Area
☐	v16.3	Fam. Hist of Breast Cancer
☐	v17.4	Fam. Hist of Cardiovasc Dis
☐	v20.2	Well Child
☐	v22.0	Pregnancy - First Normal
☐	v22.1	Pregnancy - Normal

Previous Balance	Today's Charges	Total Due	Amount Paid	New Balance
_____	_____	_____	_____	_____

Follow Up

PRN _____ Weeks _____   Months _____ Units _____

Next Appointment Date: Time:

I hereby authorize release of any information acquired in the course of examination or treatment and allow a photocopy of my signature to be used.

_____

2. Based on the information found on the encounter form, enter the procedure and diagnosis for Catherine Viajo. Compare your screen to Figure 3-4.

Figure 3-4 Procedure Entry – Viajo

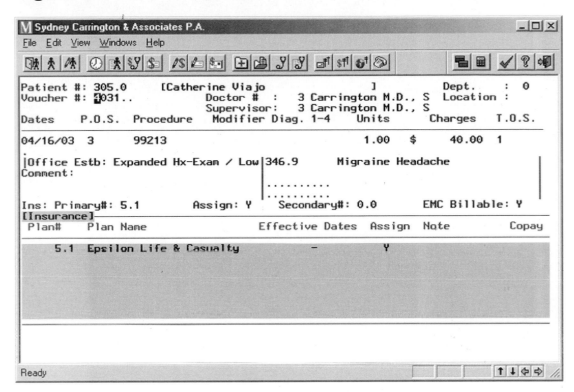

EXERCISE 3: MULTIPLE PROCEDURES, ONE DIAGNOSIS, ONE INSURANCE

JOHN WYATT

GOAL(S): In this exercise you will enter multiple procedures and a single diagnosis for a patient with insurance.

1. Before posting your entry, study the encounter form in Figure 3-5 (page 36). Answer the following questions.

   a. Who is the patient? _____

   b. What is the voucher number on the encounter form? _____

   c. Which doctor saw the patient? _____

   d. How many procedures were completed at this visit? _____

   e. How many diagnoses are listed? _____

Figure 3-5 Encounter Form – Wyatt

Sydney Carrington & Associates P.A.
34 Sycamore Street   Suite 300
Madison, CA 95653

Date: 04/16/2003

Time:

Patient: John Wyatt
Guarantor:

Voucher No.: 4032

Patient No: 307.0
Doctor: 1 - J. Monroe

	CPT	DESCRIPTION	FEE
	OFFICE/HOSPITAL CONSULTS		
☐	99201	Office New:Focused Hx-Exam	
☐	99202	Office New:Expanded Hx-Exam	
☐	99211	Office Estb:Min/None Hx-Exa	
☐	99212	Office Estb:Focused Hx-Exam	
☒	99213	Office Estb:Expanded Hx-Exa	
☐	99214	Office Estb:Detailed Hx-Exa	
☐	99215	Office Estb:Comprh Hx-Exam	
☐	99221	Hosp. Initial:Comprh Hx-	
☐	99223	Hosp.Ini:Comprh Hx-Exam/Hi	
☐	99231	Hosp. Subsequent: S-Fwd	
☐	99232	Hosp. Subsequent: Comprhn Hx	
☐	99233	Hosp. Subsequent: Ex/Hi	
☐	99238	Hospital Visit Discharge Ex	
☐	99371	Telephone Consult - Simple	
☐	99372	Telephone Consult - Intermed	
☐	99373	Telephone Consult - Complex	
☐	90843	Counseling - 25 minutes	
☐	90844	Counseling - 50 minutes	
☐	90865	Counseling - Special Interview	
	IMMUNIZATIONS/INJECTIONS		
☐	90585	BCG Vaccine	
☐	90659	Influenza Virus Vaccine	
☐	90701	Immunization-DTP	
☐	90702	DT Vaccine	
☐	90703	Tetanus Toxoids	
☐	90732	Pneumococcal Vaccine	
☐	90746	Hepatitis B Vaccine	
☐	90749	Immunization; Unlisted	

	CPT	DESCRIPTION	FEE
	LABORATORY/RADIOLOGY		
☐	81000	Urinalysis	
☐	81002	Urinalysis; Pregnancy Test	
☐	82951	Glucose Tolerance Test	
☐	84478	Triglycerides	
☐	84550	Uric Acid: Blood Chemistry	
☐	84830	Ovulation Test	
☒	85014	Hematocrit	
☒	85031	Hemogram, Complete Blood Wk	
☐	86403	Particle Agglutination Test	
☐	86485	Skin Test; Candida	
☐	86580	TB Intradermal Test	
☐	86585	TB Tine Test	
☐	87070	Culture	
☐	70190	X-Ray; Optic Foramina	
☐	70210	X-Ray Sinuses Complete	
☐	71010	Radiological Exam Ent Spine	
☐	71020	X-Ray Chest Pa & Lat	
☐	72050	X-Ray Spine, Cerv (4 views)	
☐	72090	X-Ray Spine; Scoliosis Ex	
☐	72110	Spine, lumbosacral; a/p & Lat	
☐	73030	Shoulder-Comp, min w/ 2vws	
☐	73070	Elbow, anteropost & later vws	
☐	73120	X-Ray; Hand, 2 views	
☐	73560	X-Ray, Knee, 1 or 2 views	
☐	74022	X-Ray; Abdomen, Complete	
☐	75552	Cardiac Magnetic Res Img	
☐	76020	X-Ray; Bone Age Studies	
☐	76088	Mammary Ductogram Complete	
☐	78465	Myocardial Perfusion Img	

	CPT	DESCRIPTION	FEE
	PROCEDURES/TESTS		
☐	00452	Anesthesia for Rad Surgery	
☐	11100	Skin Biopsy	
☐	15852	Dressing Change	
☐	29075	Cast Appl. - Lower Arm	
☐	29530	Strapping of Knee	
☐	29705	Removal/Revis of Cast w/Exa	
☐	53670	Catheterization Incl. Suppl	
☐	57452	Colposcopy	
☐	57505	ECC	
☐	69420	Myringotomy	
☐	92081	Visual Field Examination	
☐	92100	Serial Tonometry Exam	
☐	92120	Tonography	
☐	92552	Pure Tone Audiometry	
☐	92567	Tympanometry	
☐	93000	Electrocardiogram	
☐	93015	Exercise Stress Test (ETT)	
☐	93017	ETT Tracing Only	
☐	93040	Electrocardiogram - Rhythm	
☐	96100	Psychological Testing	
☐	99000	Specimen Handling	
☐	99058	Office Emergency Care	
☐	99070	Surgical Tray - Misc.	
☐	99080	Special Reports of Med Rec	
☐	99195	Phlebotomy	
☐			
☐			
☐			
☐			

	ICD-9 CODE DIAGNOSIS	
☐	009.0	Ill-defined Intestinal Infect
☐	133.2	Establish Baseline
☐	174.9	Breast Cancer
☐	185.0	Prostate Cancer
☐	250	Diabetes Mellitus
☐	272.4	Hyperlipidemia
☐	282.5	Anemia - Sickle Trait
☐	282.60	Anemia - Sickle Cell
☒	285.9	Anemia, Unspecified
☐	300.4	Neurotic Depression
☐	340	Multiple Sclerosis
☐	342.9	Hemiplegia - Unspecified
☐	346.9	Migraine Headache
☐	352.9	Cranial Neuralgia
☐	354.0	Carpal Tunnel Syndrome
☐	355.0	Sciatic Nerve Root Lesion
☐	366.9	Cataract
☐	386.0	Vertigo
☐	401.1	Essential Hypertension
☐	414.9	Ischemic Hearth Disease
☐	428.0	Congestive Heart Failure

	ICD-9 CODE DIAGNOSIS	
☐	435.0	Basilar Artery Syndrome
☐	440.0	Atherosclerosis
☐	442.81	Carotid Artery
☐	460.0	Common Cold
☐	461.9	Acute Sinusitis
☐	474.0	Tonsillitis
☐	477.9	Hay Fever
☐	487.0	Flu
☐	496	Chronic Airway Obstruction
☐	522	Low Red Blood Count
☐	524.6	Temporo-Mandibular Jnt Synd
☐	538.8	Stomach Pain
☐	553.3	Hiatal Hernia
☐	564.1	Spastic Colon
☐	571.4	Chronic Hepatitis
☐	571.5	Cirrhosis of Liver
☐	573.3	Hepatitis
☐	575.2	Obstruction of Gallbladder
☐	648.2	Anemia - Compl. Pregnancy
☐	715.90	Osteoarthritis - Unspec
☐	721.3	Lumbar Osteo/Spondylarthrit

	ICD-9 CODE DIAGNOSIS	
☐	724.2	Pain: Lower Back
☐	727.6	Rupture of Achilles Tendon
☐	780.1	Hallucinations
☐	780.3	Convulsions
☐	780.5	Sleep Disturbances
☐	783.0	Anorexia
☐	783.1	Abnormal Weight Gain
☐	783.2	Abnormal Weight Loss
☐	830.6	Dislocated Hip
☐	830.9	Dislocated Shoulder
☐	841.2	Sprained Wrist
☐	842.5	Sprained Ankle
☐	891.2	Fractured Tibia
☐	892.0	Fractured Fibula
☐	919.5	Insect Bite, Nonvenomous
☐	921.1	Contus Eyelid/Perioc Area
☐	v16.3	Fam. Hist of Breast Cancer
☐	v17.4	Fam. Hist of Cardiovasc Dis
☐	v20.2	Well Child
☐	v22.0	Pregnancy - First Normal
☐	v22.1	Pregnancy - Normal

Previous Balance	Today's Charges	Total Due	Amount Paid	New Balance
_____	_____	_____	_____	_____

Follow Up

PRN _____ Weeks _____ Months _____ Units _____

Next Appointment Date: _____   Time:

I hereby authorize release of any information acquired in the course of examination or treatment and allow a photocopy of my signature to be used.

2. Based on the information found on the encounter form, enter the procedures and diagnosis for John Wyatt. After you have posted all the charges, compare your screen to Figure 3-6.

Figure 3-6 Three Posted Charges – Wyatt

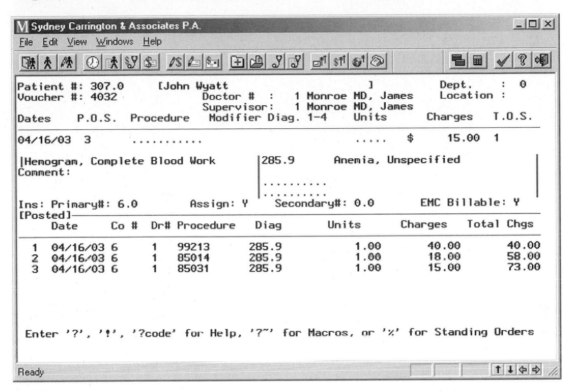

EXERCISE 4: MULTIPLE PROCEDURES WITH DIFFERENT DIAGNOSIS, MULTIPLE INSURANCE

CHRISTINE CUSACK

GOAL(S): In this exercise you will need to match procedures with different diagnoses.

1. Before posting your entry, study the encounter form in Figure 3-7 (page 40). Answer the following questions.

   a. What diagnosis would you match with the office visit? _____

   b. What diagnosis would you match with the cast application of the lower arm? _____

   c. How many procedures were completed at this visit? _____

   d. How many diagnoses are listed? _____

Figure 3-7 Encounter Form – Cusack

Sydney Carrington & Associates P.A.
34 Sycamore Street   Suite 300
Madison, CA 95653

Date: 04/16/2003

Time:

Patient: Christine Cusack
Guarantor:

Voucher No.: 4033

Patient No: 306.0
Doctor: 1 - J. Monroe

☐ CPT	DESCRIPTION	FEE
OFFICE/HOSPITAL CONSULTS		
☐ 99201	Office New:Focused Hx-Exam	
☐ 99202	Office New:Expanded Hx-Exam	
☐ 99211	Office Estb:Min/None Hx-Exa	
☐ 99212	Office Estb:Focused Hx-Exam	
☐ 99213	Office Estb:Expanded Hx-Exa	
☒ 99214	Office Estb:Detailed Hx-Exa	
☐ 99215	Office Estb:Comprhn Hx-Exam	
☐ 99221	Hosp. Initial:Comprh Hx-	
☐ 99223	Hosp.Ini:Comprh Hx-Exam/Hi	
☐ 99231	Hosp. Subsequent: S-Fwd	
☐ 99232	Hosp. Subsequent: Comprhn Hx	
☐ 99233	Hosp. Subsequent: Ex/Hi	
☐ 99238	Hospital Visit Discharge Ex	
☐ 99371	Telephone Consult - Simple	
☐ 99372	Telephone Consult - Intermed	
☐ 99373	Telephone Consult - Complex	
☐ 90843	Counseling - 25 minutes	
☐ 90844	Counseling - 50 minutes	
☐ 90865	Counseling - Special Interview	
IMMUNIZATIONS/INJECTIONS		
☐ 90585	BCG Vaccine	
☐ 90659	Influenza Virus Vaccine	
☐ 90701	Immunization-DTP	
☐ 90702	DT Vaccine	
☐ 90703	Tetanus Toxoids	
☐ 90732	Pneumococcal Vaccine	
☐ 90746	Hepatitis B Vaccine	
☐ 90749	Immunization; Unlisted	

☐ CPT	DESCRIPTION	FEE
LABORATORY/RADIOLOGY		
☐ 81000	Urinalysis	
☐ 81002	Urinalysis; Pregnancy Test	
☐ 82951	Glucose Tolerance Test	
☐ 84478	Triglycerides	
☐ 84550	Uric Acid: Blood Chemistry	
☐ 84830	Ovulation Test	
☐ 85014	Hematocrit	
☐ 85031	Hemogram, Complete Blood Wk	
☐ 86403	Particle Agglutination Test	
☐ 86485	Skin Test; Candida	
☐ 86580	TB Intradermal Test	
☐ 86585	TB Tine Test	
☐ 87070	Culture	
☐ 70190	X-Ray; Optic Foramina	
☐ 70210	X-Ray Sinuses Complete	
☐ 71010	Radiological Exam Ent Spine	
☐ 71020	X-Ray Chest Pa & Lat	
☐ 72050	X-Ray Spine, Cerv (4 views)	
☐ 72090	X-Ray Spine; Scoliosis Ex	
☐ 72110	Spine, lumbosacral; a/p & Lat	
☐ 73030	Shoulder-Comp, min w/ 2vws	
☐ 73070	Elbow, anteropost & later vws	
☐ 73120	X-Ray; Hand, 2 views	
☐ 73560	X-Ray, Knee, 1 or 2 views	
☐ 74022	X-Ray; Abdomen, Complete	
☐ 75552	Cardiac Magnetic Res Img	
☐ 76020	X-Ray; Bone Age Studies	
☐ 76088	Mammary Ductogram Complete	
☐ 78465	Myocardial Perfusion Img	

☐ CPT	DESCRIPTION	FEE
PROCEDURES/TESTS		
☐ 00452	Anesthesia for Rad Surgery	
☐ 11100	Skin Biopsy	
☐ 15852	Dressing Change	
☒ 29075	Cast Appl. - Lower Arm	
☐ 29530	Strapping of Knee	
☐ 29705	Removal/Revis of Cast w/Exa	
☐ 53670	Catheterization Incl. Suppl	
☐ 57452	Colposcopy	
☐ 57505	ECC	
☐ 69420	Myringotomy	
☐ 92081	Visual Field Examination	
☐ 92100	Serial Tonometry Exam	
☐ 92120	Tonography	
☐ 92552	Pure Tone Audiometry	
☐ 92567	Tympanometry	
☐ 93000	Electrocardiogram	
☐ 93015	Exercise Stress Test (ETT)	
☐ 93017	ETT Tracing Only	
☐ 93040	Electrocardiogram - Rhythm	
☐ 96100	Psychological Testing	
☐ 99000	Specimen Handling	
☐ 99058	Office Emergency Care	
☐ 99070	Surgical Tray - Misc.	
☐ 99080	Special Reports of Med Rec	
☐ 99195	Phlebotomy	
☐ ___	_____	
☐ ___	_____	
☐ ___	_____	

☐	ICD-9 CODE DIAGNOSIS		☐	ICD-9 CODE DIAGNOSIS		☐	ICD-9 CODE DIAGNOSIS
☐ 009.0	Ill-defined Intestinal Infect		☐ 435.0	Basilar Artery Syndrome		☐ 724.2	Pain: Lower Back
☐ 133.2	Establish Baseline		☐ 440.0	Atherosclerosis		☐ 727.6	Rupture of Achilles Tendon
☐ 174.9	Breast Cancer		☐ 442.81	Carotid Artery		☐ 780.1	Hallucinations
☐ 185.0	Prostate Cancer		☒ 460.0	Common Cold		☐ 780.3	Convulsions
☐ 250	Diabetes Mellitus		☐ 461.9	Acute Sinusitis		☐ 780.5	Sleep Disturbances
☐ 272.4	Hyperlipidemia		☐ 474.0	Tonsillitis		☐ 783.0	Anorexia
☐ 282.5	Anemia - Sickle Trait		☐ 477.9	Hay Fever		☐ 783.1	Abnormal Weight Gain
☐ 282.60	Anemia - Sickle Cell		☐ 487.0	Flu		☐ 783.2	Abnormal Weight Loss
☐ 285.9	Anemia, Unspecified		☐ 496	Chronic Airway Obstruction		☐ 830.6	Dislocated Hip
☐ 300.4	Neurotic Depression		☐ 522	Low Red Blood Count		☒ 830.9	Dislocated Shoulder
☐ 340	Multiple Sclerosis		☐ 524.6	Temporo-Mandibular Jnt Synd		☒ 841.2	Sprained Wrist
☐ 342.9	Hemiplegia - Unspecified		☐ 538.8	Stomach Pain		☐ 842.5	Sprained Ankle
☐ 346.9	Migraine Headache		☐ 553.3	Hiatal Hernia		☐ 891.2	Fractured Tibia
☐ 352.9	Cranial Neuralgia		☐ 564.1	Spastic Colon		☐ 892.0	Fractured Fibula
☐ 354.0	Carpal Tunnel Syndrome		☐ 571.4	Chronic Hepatitis		☐ 919.5	Insect Bite, Nonvenomous
☐ 355.0	Sciatic Nerve Root Lesion		☐ 571.5	Cirrhosis of Liver		☐ 921.1	Contus Eyelid/Perioc Area
☐ 366.9	Cataract		☐ 573.3	Hepatitis		☐ v16.3	Fam. Hist of Breast Cancer
☐ 386.0	Vertigo		☐ 575.2	Obstruction of Gallbladder		☐ v17.4	Fam. Hist of Cardiovasc Dis
☐ 401.1	Essential Hypertension		☐ 648.2	Anemia - Compl. Pregnancy		☐ v20.2	Well Child
☐ 414.9	Ischemic Hearth Disease		☐ 715.90	Osteoarthritis - Unspec		☐ v22.0	Pregnancy - First Normal
☐ 428.0	Congestive Heart Failure		☐ 721.3	Lumbar Osteo/Spondylarthrit		☐ v22.1	Pregnancy - Normal

Previous Balance	Today's Charges	Total Due	Amount Paid	New Balance
_____	_____	_____	_____	_____

Follow Up

PRN _____ Weeks _____ Months _____ Units _____

Next Appointment Date: Time:

I hereby authorize release of any information acquired in the course of examination or treatment and allow a photocopy of my signature to be used.

_____

2. Based on the information found on the encounter form, enter the procedures and diagnoses for Christine Cusack. After posting both charges, compare your screen to Figure 3-8.

Figure 3-8 Two Procedures Posted – Cusack

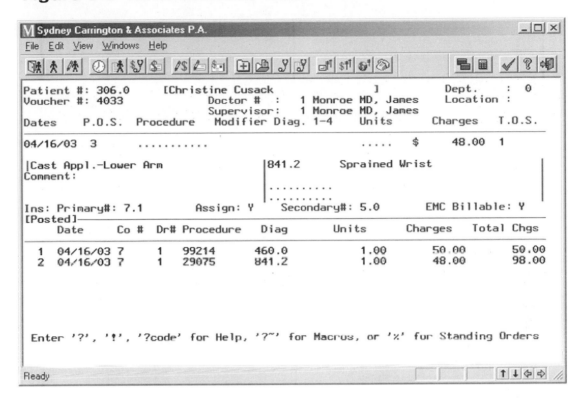

EXERCISE 5: MULTIPLE PROCEDURES, ONE DIAGNOSIS, ONE INSURANCE FOR PATIENT WITH DIFFERENT LAST NAME

MATTHEW NOONAN

GOAL(S): In this exercise you will enter procedures and a diagnosis for a patient with a different last name than the guarantor.

1. Before posting your entry, study the encounter form in Figure 3-9 (page 44). Answer the following questions.

   a. Who is the patient? _____

   b. How will you need to search for this patient that has a different last name than the guarantor?

   _____

   d. How many procedures were completed at this visit? _____

   e. How many diagnoses are listed? _____

Figure 3-9 Encounter Form – Noonan

Sydney Carrington & Associates P.A.
34 Sycamore Street   Suite 300
Madison, CA 95653

Date: 04/16/2003   Voucher No.:   4034

Time:

Patient: Matthew Noonan   Patient No: 310.1
Guarantor: Doctor: 2 - F. Simpson

CPT	DESCRIPTION	FEE
OFFICE/HOSPITAL CONSULTS		
☐ 99201	Office New:Focused Hx-Exam	
☐ 99202	Office New:Expanded Hx-Exam	
☐ 99211	Office Estb:Min/None Hx-Exa	
☐ 99212	Office Estb:Focused Hx-Exam	
☒ 99213	Office Estb:Expanded Hx-Exa	
☐ 99214	Office Estb:Detailed Hx-Exa	
☐ 99215	Office Estb:Comprhn Hx-Exam	
☐ 99221	Hosp. Initial:Comprh Hx-	
☐ 99223	Hosp.Ini:Comprh Hx-Exam/Hi	
☐ 99231	Hosp. Subsequent: S-Fwd	
☐ 99232	Hosp. Subsequent: Comprhn Hx	
☐ 99233	Hosp. Subsequent: Ex/Hi	
☐ 99238	Hospital Visit Discharge Ex	
☐ 99371	Telephone Consult - Simple	
☐ 99372	Telephone Consult - Intermed	
☐ 99373	Telephone Consult - Complex	
☐ 90843	Counseling - 25 minutes	
☒ 90844	Counseling - 50 minutes	
☐ 90865	Counseling - Special Interview	
IMMUNIZATIONS/INJECTIONS		
☐ 90585	BCG Vaccine	
☐ 90659	Influenza Virus Vaccine	
☐ 90701	Immunization-DTP	
☐ 90702	DT Vaccine	
☐ 90703	Tetanus Toxoids	
☐ 90732	Pneumococcal Vaccine	
☐ 90746	Hepatitis B Vaccine	
☐ 90749	Immunization; Unlisted	

CPT	DESCRIPTION	FEE
LABORATORY/RADIOLOGY		
☐ 81000	Urinalysis	
☐ 81002	Urinalysis; Pregnancy Test	
☐ 82951	Glucose Tolerance Test	
☐ 84478	Triglycerides	
☐ 84550	Uric Acid: Blood Chemistry	
☐ 84830	Ovulation Test	
☐ 85014	Hematocrit	
☐ 85031	Hemogram, Complete Blood Wk	
☐ 86403	Particle Agglutination Test	
☐ 86485	Skin Test; Candida	
☐ 86580	TB Intradermal Test	
☐ 86585	TB Tine Test	
☐ 87070	Culture	
☐ 70190	X-Ray; Optic Foramina	
☐ 70210	X-Ray Sinuses Complete	
☐ 71010	Radiological Exam Ent Spine	
☐ 71020	X-Ray Chest Pa & Lat	
☐ 72050	X-Ray Spine, Cerv (4 views)	
☐ 72090	X-Ray Spine; Scoliosis Ex	
☐ 72110	Spine, lumbosacral; a/p & Lat	
☐ 73030	Shoulder-Comp, min w/ 2vws	
☐ 73070	Elbow, anteropost & later vws	
☐ 73120	X-Ray; Hand, 2 views	
☐ 73560	X-Ray, Knee, 1 or 2 views	
☐ 74022	X-Ray; Abdomen, Complete	
☐ 75552	Cardiac Magnetic Res Img	
☐ 76020	X-Ray; Bone Age Studies	
☐ 76088	Mammary Ductogram Complete	
☐ 78465	Myocardial Perfusion Img	

CPT	DESCRIPTION	FEE
PROCEDURES/TESTS		
☐ 00452	Anesthesia for Rad Surgery	
☐ 11100	Skin Biopsy	
☐ 15852	Dressing Change	
☐ 29075	Cast Appl. - Lower Arm	
☐ 29530	Strapping of Knee	
☐ 29705	Removal/Revis of Cast w/Exa	
☐ 53670	Catheterization Incl. Suppl	
☐ 57452	Colposcopy	
☐ 57505	ECC	
☐ 69420	Myringotomy	
☐ 92081	Visual Field Examination	
☐ 92100	Serial Tonometry Exam	
☐ 92120	Tonography	
☐ 92552	Pure Tone Audiometry	
☐ 92567	Tympanometry	
☐ 93000	Electrocardiogram	
☐ 93015	Exercise Stress Test (ETT)	
☐ 93017	ETT Tracing Only	
☐ 93040	Electrocardiogram - Rhythm	
☐ 96100	Psychological Testing	
☐ 99000	Specimen Handling	
☐ 99058	Office Emergency Care	
☐ 99070	Surgical Tray - Misc.	
☐ 99080	Special Reports of Med Rec	
☐ 99195	Phlebotomy	
☐ _____	_____	
☐ _____	_____	
☐ _____	_____	

ICD-9 CODE DIAGNOSIS		
☐ 009.0	Ill-defined Intestinal Infect	
☐ 133.2	Establish Baseline	
☐ 174.9	Breast Cancer	
☐ 185.0	Prostate Cancer	
☐ 250	Diabetes Mellitus	
☐ 272.4	Hyperlipidemia	
☐ 282.5	Anemia - Sickle Trait	
☐ 282.60	Anemia - Sickle Cell	
☐ 285.9	Anemia, Unspecified	
☐ 300.4	Neurotic Depression	
☐ 340	Multiple Sclerosis	
☐ 342.9	Hemiplegia - Unspecified	
☐ 346.9	Migraine Headache	
☐ 352.9	Cranial Neuralgia	
☐ 354.0	Carpal Tunnel Syndrome	
☐ 355	Sciatic Nerve Root Lesion	
☐ 366.9	Cataract	
☐ 386.0	Vertigo	
☐ 401.1	Essential Hypertension	
☐ 414.9	Ischemic Hearth Disease	
☐ 428.0	Congestive Heart Failure	

ICD-9 CODE DIAGNOSIS		
☐ 435.0	Basilar Artery Syndrome	
☐ 440.0	Atherosclerosis	
☐ 442.81	Carotid Artery	
☐ 460.0	Common Cold	
☐ 461.9	Acute Sinusitis	
☐ 474.0	Tonsillitis	
☐ 477.9	Hay Fever	
☐ 487.0	Flu	
☐ 496	Chronic Airway Obstruction	
☐ 522	Low Red Blood Count	
☐ 524.6	Temporo-Mandibular Jnt Synd	
☐ 538.8	Stomach Pain	
☐ 553.3	Hiatal Hernia	
☐ 564.1	Spastic Colon	
☐ 571.4	Chronic Hepatitis	
☐ 571.5	Cirrhosis of Liver	
☐ 573.3	Hepatitis	
☐ 575.2	Obstruction of Gallbladder	
☐ 648.2	Anemia - Compl. Pregnancy	
☐ 715.90	Osteoarthritis - Unspec	
☐ 721.3	Lumbar Osteo/Spondylarthrit	

ICD-9 CODE DIAGNOSIS		
☐ 724.2	Pain: Lower Back	
☐ 727.6	Rupture of Achilles Tendon	
☐ 780.1	Hallucinations	
☐ 780.3	Convulsions	
☒ 780.5	Sleep Disturbances	
☐ 783.0	Anorexia	
☐ 783.1	Abnormal Weight Gain	
☐ 783.2	Abnormal Weight Loss	
☐ 830.6	Dislocated Hip	
☐ 830.9	Dislocated Shoulder	
☐ 841.2	Sprained Wrist	
☐ 842.5	Sprained Ankle	
☐ 891.2	Fractured Tibia	
☐ 892.0	Fractured Fibula	
☐ 919.5	Insect Bite, Nonvenomous	
☐ 921.1	Contus Eyelid/Perioc Area	
☐ v16.3	Fam. Hist of Breast Cancer	
☐ v17.4	Fam. Hist of Cardiovasc Dis	
☐ v20.2	Well Child	
☐ v22.0	Pregnancy - First Normal	
☐ v22.1	Pregnancy - Normal	

Previous Balance	Today's Charges	Total Due	Amount Paid	New Balance
_____	_____	_____	_____	_____

Follow Up

PRN _____ Weeks _____   Months _____ Units _____

Next Appointment Date: Time:

I hereby authorize release of any information acquired in the course of
examination or treatment and allow a photocopy of my signature to be used.

_____   _____

2. Based on the information found on the encounter form, enter the procedures and diagnoses for Matthew Noonan. After posting the procedures, compare your screen to Figure 3-10.

Figure 3-10   Two Procedures Posted – Noonan

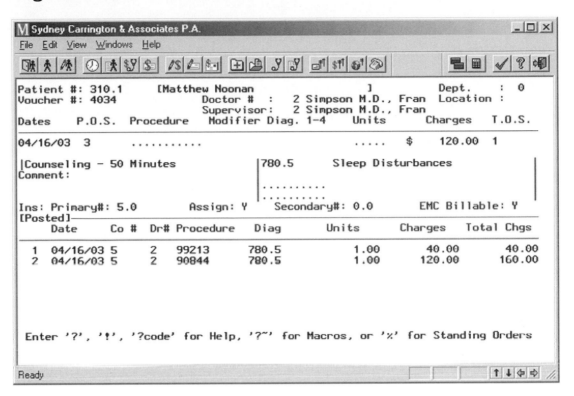

EXERCISE 6: WORKER'S COMPENSATION WITH AILMENT

ROBERTO VEGA

GOAL(S): In this exercise you will enter procedures and a diagnosis for a patient that was hurt at work. Since this is a worker's compensation case, you will need to add Ailment Detail for the insurance company.

1. Before posting your entry, study the encounter form in Figure 3-11 (page 48). Answer the following questions.

   a. Who is the patient? _____

   b. How many procedures were completed at this visit? _____

   c. After adding the Ailment Detail for the first procedure, what response to Ailment Detail is entered for the remaining procedures? _____

   e. How many diagnoses are listed? _____

Figure 3-11 Encounter Form – Vega

Sydney Carrington & Associates P.A.
34 Sycamore Street   Suite 300
Madison, CA 95653

Date: 04/16/2003

Voucher No.: 4035

Time:

Patient: Roberto Vega
Guarantor:

Patient No: 311.1
Doctor: 1 - J. Monroe

CPT	DESCRIPTION	FEE	CPT	DESCRIPTION	FEE	CPT	DESCRIPTION	FEE
OFFICE/HOSPITAL CONSULTS			**LABORATORY/RADIOLOGY**			**PROCEDURES/TESTS**		
☐ 99201	Office New:Focused Hx-Exam		☐ 81000	Urinalysis		☐ 00452	Anesthesia for Rad Surgery	
☐ 99202	Office New:Expanded Hx-Exam		☐ 81002	Urinalysis; Pregnancy Test		☐ 11100	Skin Biopsy	
☐ 99211	Office Estb:Min/None Hx-Exa		☐ 82951	Glucose Tolerance Test		☐ 15852	Dressing Change	
☐ 99212	Office Estb:Focused Hx-Exam		☐ 84478	Triglycerides		☐ 29075	Cast Appl. - Lower Arm	
☐ 99213	Office Estb:Expanded Hx-Exa		☐ 84550	Uric Acid: Blood Chemistry		☐ 29530	Strapping of Knee	
☒ 99214	Office Estb:Detailed Hx-Exa		☐ 84830	Ovulation Test		☐ 29705	Removal/Revis of Cast w/Exa	
☐ 99215	Office Estb:Comprhn Hx-Exam		☐ 85014	Hematocrit		☐ 53670	Catheterization Incl. Suppl	
☐ 99221	Hosp. Initial:Comprh Hx-		☐ 85031	Hemogram, Complete Blood Wk		☐ 57452	Colposcopy	
☐ 99223	Hosp.Ini:Comprh Hx-Exam/Hi		☐ 86403	Particle Agglutination Test		☐ 57505	ECC	
☐ 99231	Hosp. Subsequent: S-Fwd		☐ 86485	Skin Test; Candida		☐ 69420	Myringotomy	
☐ 99232	Hosp. Subsequent: Comprhn Hx		☐ 86580	TB Intradermal Test		☐ 92081	Visual Field Examination	
☐ 99233	Hosp. Subsequent: Ex/Hi		☐ 86585	TB Tine Test		☐ 92100	Serial Tonometry Exam	
☐ 99238	Hospital Visit Discharge Ex		☐ 87070	Culture		☐ 92120	Tonography	
☐ 99371	Telephone Consult - Simple		☐ 70190	X-Ray; Optic Foramina		☐ 92552	Pure Tone Audiometry	
☐ 99372	Telephone Consult - Intermed		☐ 70210	X-Ray Sinuses Complete		☐ 92567	Tympanometry	
☐ 99373	Telephone Consult - Complex		☐ 71010	Radiological Exam Ent Spine		☐ 93000	Electrocardiogram	
☐ 90843	Counseling - 25 minutes		☐ 71020	X-Ray Chest Pa & Lat		☐ 93015	Exercise Stress Test (ETT)	
☐ 90844	Counseling - 50 minutes		☒ 72050	X-Ray Spine, Cerv (4 views)		☐ 93017	ETT Tracing Only	
☐ 90865	Counseling - Special Interview		☐ 72090	X-Ray Spine; Scoliosis Ex		☐ 93040	Electrocardiogram - Rhythm	
			☐ 72110	Spine, lumbosacral; a/p & Lat		☐ 96100	Psychological Testing	
IMMUNIZATIONS/INJECTIONS			☐ 73030	Shoulder-Comp, min w/ 2vws		☐ 99000	Specimen Handling	
☐ 90585	BCG Vaccine		☐ 73070	Elbow, anteropost & later vws		☐ 99058	Office Emergency Care	
☐ 90659	Influenza Virus Vaccine		☐ 73120	X-Ray; Hand, 2 views		☐ 99070	Surgical Tray - Misc.	
☐ 90701	Immunization-DTP		☐ 73560	X-Ray, Knee, 1 or 2 views		☐ 99080	Special Reports of Med Rec	
☐ 90702	DT Vaccine		☐ 74022	X-Ray; Abdomen, Complete		☐ 99195	Phlebotomy	
☐ 90703	Tetanus Toxoids		☐ 75552	Cardiac Magnetic Res Img		☐		
☐ 90732	Pneumococcal Vaccine		☐ 76020	X-Ray; Bone Age Studies		☐		
☐ 90746	Hepatitis B Vaccine		☐ 76088	Mammary Ductogram Complete		☐		
☐ 90749	Immunization; Unlisted		☐ 78465	Myocardial Perfusion Img				

	ICD-9 CODE DIAGNOSIS			ICD-9 CODE DIAGNOSIS			ICD-9 CODE DIAGNOSIS	
☐	009.0	Ill-defined Intestinal Infect	☐	435.0	Basilar Artery Syndrome	☒	724.2	Pain: Lower Back
☐	133.2	Establish Baseline	☐	440.0	Atherosclerosis	☐	727.6	Rupture of Achilles Tendon
☐	174.9	Breast Cancer	☐	442.81	Carotid Artery	☐	780.1	Hallucinations
☐	185.0	Prostate Cancer	☐	460.0	Common Cold	☐	780.3	Convulsions
☐	250	Diabetes Mellitus	☐	461.9	Acute Sinusitis	☐	780.5	Sleep Disturbances
☐	272.4	Hyperlipidemia	☐	474.0	Tonsillitis	☐	783.0	Anorexia
☐	282.5	Anemia - Sickle Trait	☐	477.9	Hay Fever	☐	783.1	Abnormal Weight Gain
☐	282.60	Anemia - Sickle Cell	☐	487.0	Flu	☐	783.2	Abnormal Weight Loss
☐	285.9	Anemia, Unspecified	☐	496	Chronic Airway Obstruction	☐	830.6	Dislocated Hip
☐	300.4	Neurotic Depression	☐	522	Low Red Blood Count	☐	830.9	Dislocated Shoulder
☐	340	Multiple Sclerosis	☐	524.6	Temporo-Mandibular Jnt Synd	☐	841.2	Sprained Wrist
☐	342.9	Hemiplegia - Unspecified	☐	538.8	Stomach Pain	☐	842.5	Sprained Ankle
☐	346.9	Migraine Headache	☐	553.3	Hiatal Hernia	☐	891.2	Fractured Tibia
☐	352.9	Cranial Neuralgia	☐	564.1	Spastic Colon	☐	892.0	Fractured Fibula
☐	354.0	Carpal Tunnel Syndrome	☐	571.4	Chronic Hepatitis	☐	919.5	Insect Bite, Nonvenomous
☐	355.0	Sciatic Nerve Root Lesion	☐	571.5	Cirrhosis of Liver	☐	921.1	Contus Eyelid/Perioc Area
☐	366.9	Cataract	☐	573.0	Hepatitis	☐	v16.3	Fam. Hist of Breast Cancer
☐	386.0	Vertigo	☐	575.2	Obstruction of Gallbladder	☐	v17.4	Fam. Hist of Cardiovasc Dis
☐	401.1	Essential Hypertension	☐	648.2	Anemia - Compl. Pregnancy	☐	v20.2	Well Child
☐	414.9	Ischemic Hearth Disease	☐	715.90	Osteoarthritis - Unspec	☐	v22.0	Pregnancy - First Normal
☐	428.0	Congestive Heart Failure	☐	721.3	Lumbar Osteo/Spondylarthrit	☐	v22.1	Pregnancy - Normal

Previous Balance	Today's Charges	Total Due	Amount Paid	New Balance
_____	_____	_____	_____	_____

Follow Up

PRN _____ Weeks _____ Months _____ Units _____

Next Appointment Date: Time:

I hereby authorize release of any information acquired in the course of
examination or treatment and allow a photocopy of my signature to be used.

_____

2. Based on the information found on the encounter form, enter the procedures and diagnosis for Roberto Vega. When prompted for Ailment Detail, use the following information to complete the Ailment Detail screen (accept default response if not indicated):

Hold Claim: (N)ormal Billing

Date First Consulted: 04/16/03

Comment Field: WC Back

Related to Employment: (Y)es

Accident: (W)ork

Old Symptom: (N)o

Emergency: (N)o

Date of first symptom: 04/16/03

Date resumed work: 04/17/03

Dates of Disability (Partial): 04/16/03 to (LEAVE BLANK)

Compare your screens to Figures 3-12 and 3-13.

Figure 3-12 Ailment Detail – Vega

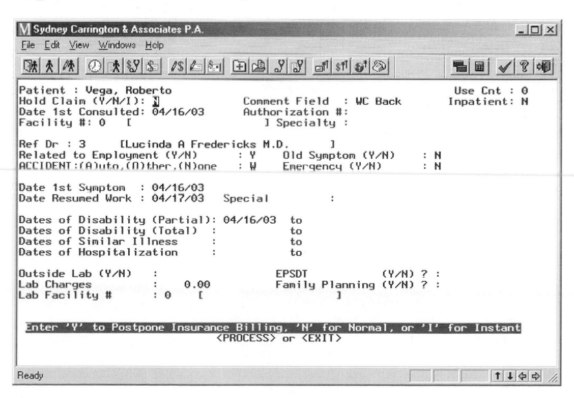

Figure 3-13 Two Procedures Posted – Vega

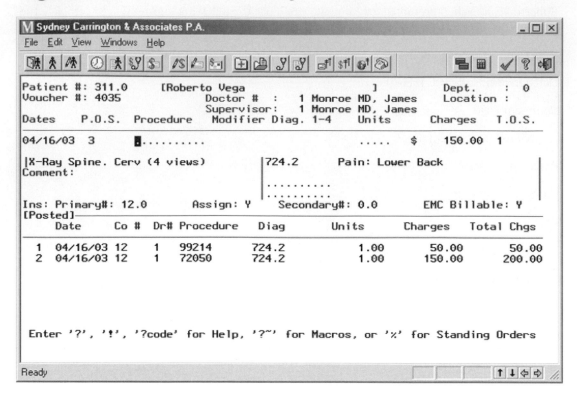

EXERCISE 7: WORK-INS

LINDA FROST

GOAL(S): In this exercise you will enter procedures and a diagnosis for a patient who does not have a preprinted encounter form.

1. Before posting your entry, study the encounter form in Figure 3-14 (page 52). Answer the following questions.

   a. Who is the patient? _____

   b. What will you enter for the voucher number? _____

   d. How many procedures were completed at this visit? _____

   e. How many diagnoses are listed? _____

Figure 3-14 Encounter Form – Frost

Sydney Carrington & Associates P.A.
34 Sycamore Street Suite 300
Madison, CA 95653

Date: 04/16/2003

Time:

Patient: Linda Frost
Guarantor:

Voucher No.: Work-In

Patient No: 308.1
Doctor: 3 - S. Carrington

OFFICE/HOSPITAL CONSULTS

CPT	DESCRIPTION	FEE
☐ 99201	Office New:Focused Hx-Exam	
☐ 99202	Office New:Expanded Hx-Exam	
☐ 99211	Office Estb:Min/None Hx-Exa	
☐ 99212	Office Estb:Focused Hx-Exam	
☒ 99213	Office Estb:Expanded Hx-Exa	
☐ 99214	Office Estb:Detailed Hx-Exa	
☐ 99215	Office Estb:Comprhn Hx-Exam	
☐ 99221	Hosp. Initial:Comprh Hx-	
☐ 99223	Hosp.Ini:Comprh Hx-Exam/Hi	
☐ 99231	Hosp. Subsequent: S-Fwd	
☐ 99232	Hosp. Subsequent: Comprhn Hx	
☐ 99233	Hosp. Subsequent: Ex/Hi	
☐ 99238	Hospital Visit Discharge Ex	
☐ 99371	Telephone Consult - Simple	
☐ 99372	Telephone Consult - Intermed	
☐ 99373	Telephone Consult - Complex	
☐ 90843	Counseling - 25 minutes	
☐ 90844	Counseling - 50 minutes	
☐ 90865	Counseling - Special Interview	

IMMUNIZATIONS/INJECTIONS

CPT	DESCRIPTION	FEE
☐ 90585	BCG Vaccine	
☐ 90659	Influenza Virus Vaccine	
☐ 90701	Immunization-DTP	
☐ 90702	DT Vaccine	
☐ 90703	Tetanus Toxoids	
☐ 90732	Pneumococcal Vaccine	
☐ 90746	Hepatitis B Vaccine	
☐ 90749	Immunization; Unlisted	

LABORATORY/RADIOLOGY

CPT	DESCRIPTION	FEE
☐ 81000	Urinalysis	
☐ 81002	Urinalysis; Pregnancy Test	
☐ 82951	Glucose Tolerance Test	
☐ 84478	Triglycerides	
☐ 84550	Uric Acid: Blood Chemistry	
☐ 84830	Ovulation Test	
☐ 85014	Hematocrit	
☐ 85031	Hemogram, Complete Blood Wk	
☐ 86403	Particle Agglutination Test	
☐ 86485	Skin Test; Candida	
☐ 86580	TB Intradermal Test	
☐ 86585	TB Tine Test	
☒ 87070	Culture	
☐ 70190	X-Ray; Optic Foramina	
☐ 70210	X-Ray Sinuses Complete	
☐ 71010	Radiological Exam Ent Spine	
☐ 71020	X-Ray Chest Pa & Lat	
☐ 72050	X-Ray Spine, Cerv (4 views)	
☐ 72090	X-Ray Spine; Scoliosis Ex	
☐ 72110	Spine, lumbosacral; a/p & Lat	
☐ 73030	Shoulder-Comp, min w/ 2vws	
☐ 73070	Elbow, anteropost & later vws	
☐ 73120	X-Ray; Hand, 2 views	
☐ 73560	X-Ray, Knee, 1 or 2 views	
☐ 74022	X-Ray; Abdomen, Complete	
☐ 75552	Cardiac Magnetic Res Img	
☐ 76020	X-Ray; Bone Age Studies	
☐ 76088	Mammary Ductogram Complete	
☐ 78465	Myocardial Perfusion Img	

PROCEDURES/TESTS

CPT	DESCRIPTION	FEE
☐ 00452	Anesthesia for Rad Surgery	
☐ 11100	Skin Biopsy	
☐ 15852	Dressing Change	
☐ 29075	Cast Appl. - Lower Arm	
☐ 29530	Strapping of Knee	
☐ 29705	Removal/Revis of Cast w/Exa	
☐ 53670	Catheterization Incl. Suppl	
☐ 57452	Colposcopy	
☐ 57505	ECC	
☐ 69420	Myringotomy	
☐ 92081	Visual Field Examination	
☐ 92100	Serial Tonometry Exam	
☐ 92120	Tonography	
☐ 92552	Pure Tone Audiometry	
☐ 92567	Tympanometry	
☐ 93000	Electrocardiogram	
☐ 93015	Exercise Stress Test (ETT)	
☐ 93017	ETT Tracing Only	
☐ 93040	Electrocardiogram - Rhythm	
☐ 96100	Psychological Testing	
☐ 99000	Specimen Handling	
☐ 99058	Office Emergency Care	
☐ 99070	Surgical Tray - Misc.	
☐ 99080	Special Reports of Med Rec	
☐ 99195	Phlebotomy	
☐		
☐		
☐		

ICD-9 CODE DIAGNOSIS

☐ 009.0	Ill-defined Intestinal Infect	☐ 435.0	Basilar Artery Syndrome	☒ 724.2	Pain: Lower Back
☐ 133.2	Establish Baseline	☐ 440.0	Atherosclerosis	☐ 727.6	Rupture of Achilles Tendon
☐ 174.9	Breast Cancer	☐ 442.81	Carotid Artery	☐ 780.1	Hallucinations
☐ 185.0	Prostate Cancer	☐ 460.0	Common Cold	☐ 780.3	Convulsions
☐ 250	Diabetes Mellitus	☐ 461.9	Acute Sinusitis	☐ 780.5	Sleep Disturbances
☐ 272.4	Hyperlipidemia	☒ 474.0	Tonsillitis	☐ 783.0	Anorexia
☐ 282.5	Anemia - Sickle Trait	☐ 477.9	Hay Fever	☐ 783.1	Abnormal Weight Gain
☐ 282.60	Anemia - Sickle Cell	☐ 487.0	Flu	☐ 783.2	Abnormal Weight Loss
☐ 285.9	Anemia, Unspecified	☐ 496	Chronic Airway Obstruction	☐ 830.6	Dislocated Hip
☐ 300.4	Neurotic Depression	☐ 522	Low Red Blood Count	☐ 830.9	Dislocated Shoulder
☐ 340	Multiple Sclerosis	☐ 524.6	Temporo-Mandibular Jnt Synd	☐ 841.2	Sprained Wrist
☐ 342.9	Hemiplegia - Unspecified	☐ 538.8	Stomach Pain	☐ 842.5	Sprained Ankle
☐ 346.9	Migraine Headache	☐ 553.3	Hiatal Hernia	☐ 891.2	Fractured Tibia
☐ 352.9	Cranial Neuralgia	☐ 564.1	Spastic Colon	☐ 892.0	Fractured Fibula
☐ 354.0	Carpal Tunnel Syndrome	☐ 571.4	Chronic Hepatitis	☐ 919.5	Insect Bite, Nonvenomous
☐ 355.0	Sciatic Nerve Root Lesion	☐ 571.5	Cirrhosis of Liver	☐ 921.1	Contus Eyelid/Perioc Area
☐ 366.9	Cataract	☐ 573.3	Hepatitis	☐ v16.3	Fam. Hist of Breast Cancer
☐ 386.0	Vertigo	☐ 575.2	Obstruction of Gallbladder	☐ v17.4	Fam. Hist of Cardiovasc Dis
☐ 401.1	Essential Hypertension	☐ 648.2	Anemia - Compl. Pregnancy	☐ v20.2	Well Child
☐ 414.9	Ischemic Hearth Disease	☐ 715.90	Osteoarthritis - Unspec	☐ v22.0	Pregnancy - First Normal
☐ 428.0	Congestive Heart Failure	☐ 721.3	Lumbar Osteo/Spondylarthrit	☐ v22.1	Pregnancy - Normal

Previous Balance	Today's Charges	Total Due	Amount Paid	New Balance

Follow Up
PRN _____ Weeks _____ Months _____ Units _____
Next Appointment Date: _____ Time: _____

I hereby authorize release of any information acquired in the course of examination or treatment and allow a photocopy of my signature to be used.

2. Based on the information found on the encounter form, enter the procedures and diagnosis for Linda Frost. After posting all charges, compare your screen to Figure 3-15.

Figure 3-15 Two Procedures Posted – Frost

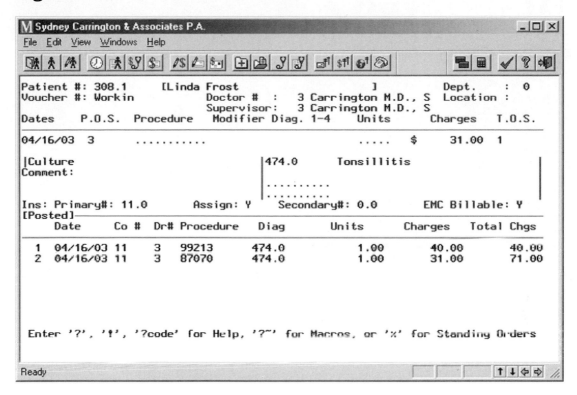

U N I T 4

Editing Prior Entries

In the unit exercises that follow, you will use the information provided to make changes to patient accounts.

EXERCISE 1: ADDING A DEPENDENT

WILLIAM SALVANI; ACCOUNT 312

GOAL(S): In this exercise you will add a dependent to an existing account.

1. Before posting your entry, study the patient registration form in Figure 4-1 (page 56). Answer the following questions:

   a. What is the relationship of the dependent to the guarantor? _____

   b. Does the dependent have extended information? _____

   c. Does the dependent have insurance? _____

Figure 4-1 Patient Registration Form – Kyle Salvani

Patient Registration Form

Sydney Carrington & Associates
34 Sycamore Street ● Madison, CA 95653

TODAY'S DATE: _04/16/2003_

FOR OFFICE USE ONLY	
ACCOUNT NO.:	312
DOCTOR:	#2
BILL TYPE:	11
EXTENDED INFO.:	0

PATIENT INFORMATION

Salvani	Kyle	M.
PATIENT LAST NAME	FIRST NAME	MI

Son
RELATIONSHIP TO GUARANTOR

M	07/09/2002	Single	214-86-1392
SEX (M/F)	DATE OF BIRTH	MARITAL STATUS	SOC. SEC. #

Floral City High School
EMPLOYER OR SCHOOL NAME

ADDRESS OF EMPLOYER OR SCHOOL

CITY	STATE	ZIP CODE

	Thomas Bennett, MD
EMPLOYER OR SCHOOL PHONE	REFERRED BY

E-MAIL

GUARANTOR INFORMATION

Salvani	William	M
RESPONSIBLE PARTY LAST NAME	FIRST NAME	MI SEX (M/F)

82 Cedar Brook Road - Apt 5A
MAILING ADDRESS   STREET ADDRESS (IF DIFFERENT)

Sacramento	CA	94056
CITY	STATE	ZIP CODE

(917) 826-1314	(917) 391-2873
(AREA CODE) HOME PHONE	(AREA CODE) WORK PHONE

02/26/1968	Married	158-23-4613
DATE OF BIRTH	MARITAL STATUS	SOC. SEC. #

Better Business Bureau
EMPLOYER NAME

EMPLOYER ADDRESS

Sacramento	CA	94056
CITY	STATE	ZIP CODE

PRIMARY INSURANCE

Epsilon Life & Casualty
NAME OF PRIMARY INSURANCE COMPANY

P.O. Box 189
ADDRESS

Macon	GA	31298
CITY	STATE	ZIP CODE

17398QX	2003BR
IDENTIFICATION #	GROUP NAME AND/OR #

William Salvani
INSURED PERSON'S NAME (IF DIFFERENT FROM THE RESPONSIBLE PARTY)

Same
ADDRESS (IF DIFFERENT)

Same

CITY	STATE	ZIP CODE

(800) 908-7654	158-23-4613
PRIMARY INSURANCE PHONE NUMBER	SOC. SEC. #

Self
WHAT IS THE RESPONSIBLE PARTY'S RELATIONSHIP TO THE INSURED?

SECONDARY INSURANCE

NAME OF SECONDARY INSURANCE COMPANY

ADDRESS

CITY	STATE	ZIP CODE

IDENTIFICATION #	GROUP NAME AND/OR #

INSURED PERSON'S NAME (IF DIFFERENT FROM THE RESPONSIBLE PARTY)

ADDRESS (IF DIFFERENT)

CITY	STATE	ZIP CODE

SECONDARY INSURANCE PHONE NUMBER	SOC. SEC. #

WHAT IS THE RESPONSIBLE PARTY'S RELATIONSHIP TO THE INSURED?

I hereby consent for Sydney Carrington & Associates, P.A. to use or disclose my health information to carry out treatment, payment, and health care operations. I authorize the use of this signature on all insurance submissions. I understand that I am financially responsible for all charges whether or not paid by the insurance. I acknowledge receipt of the practice's privacy policy.

William Salvani (father)	4/16/2003
PATIENT SIGNATURE	DATE

2. Based on the information found on the patient registration form (Figure 4-1), add the dependent to Account 312. Compare your screen to Figure 4-2.

Figure 4-2 Dependent Screen – Salvani

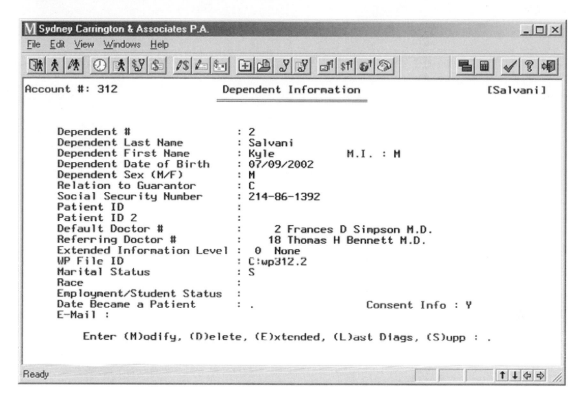

EXERCISE 2: CHANGING A GUARANTOR'S LAST NAME, ADDING AN INSURANCE POLICY

ERIN KANTOR; ACCOUNT 313

Erin Kantor is an established patient. She has recently been married and called the office to update her account information.

GOAL(S): In this exercise you will use the information provided to change a patient's last name and marital status and add insurance.

1. Erin's married name is **Stein**.

2. Modify her marital status. Compare your screen to Figure 4-3.

3. Add **Pan American** as the insurance company. Her husband, Charles Stein, is the insured person. The insurance ID # and insured party ID # is 149187341. The group number is 648N. Charles and Erin reside at 30 Wilbur Street, Woodside, CA 98076. Charles's insurance coverage is through his employer, Statton Realty. Compare your screen to Figure 4-4.

4. (S)et Coverage Priority after adding the insurance. Compare your screen to Figure 4-5.

Figure 4-3   Account Information – Stein

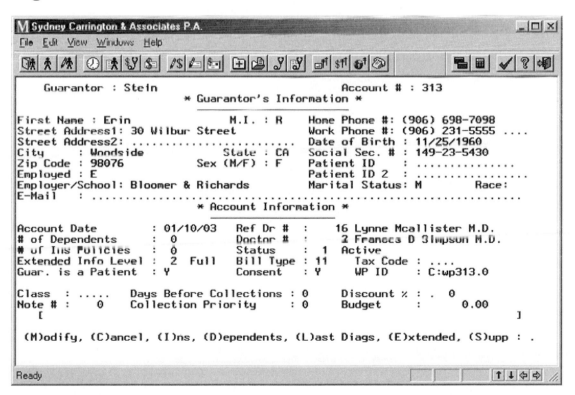

NOTE: Insured party numbers are assigned by the computer. The number assigned in this exercise may vary from that shown in Figure 4-4.

Figure 4-4 Insurance Policy – Stein

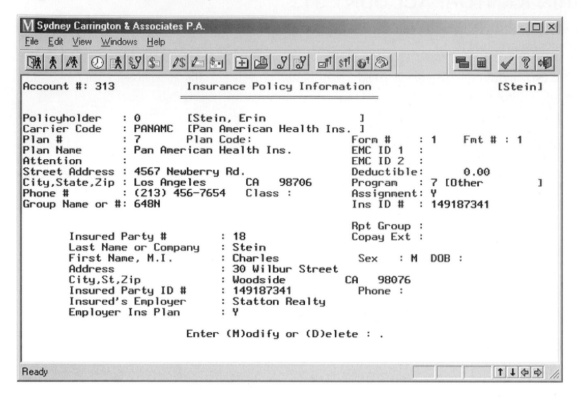

Figure 4-5 Coverage List – Stein

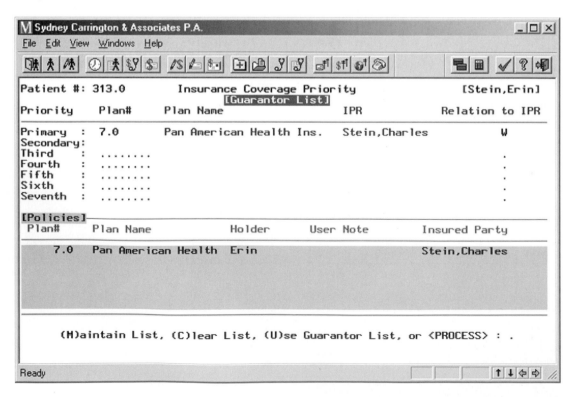

EXERCISE 3: CHANGING A GUARANTOR'S ADDRESS, EMPLOYER, AND EXTENDED INFORMATION

CARMEN FUENTAS; ACCOUNT 314

Carmen Fuentas calls to say she has moved and changed her employment.

GOAL(S): Using the information she provides, you will update her address, employment information, and telephone numbers.

1. Carmen has moved to 83 Hyatt Court, Madison, CA 95653.

2. Carmen now works at Regency Enterprises, 632 Walton Avenue, Madison, CA 95653.

3. Carmen's home phone number is (916) 810-4385. Her work phone number is (916) 539-2810. Compare your screen to Figures 4-6 and 4-7.

Figure 4-6 Account Information – Fuentas

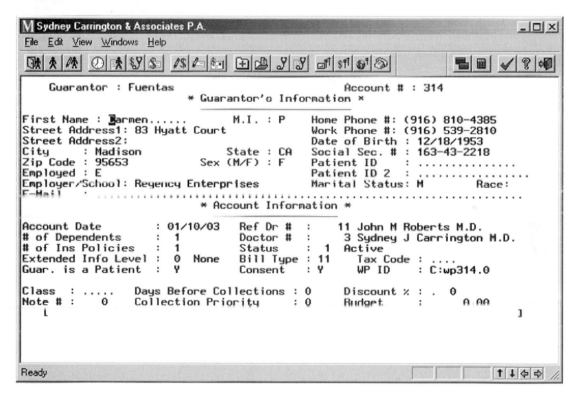

Figure 4-7 Extended Information – Fuentas

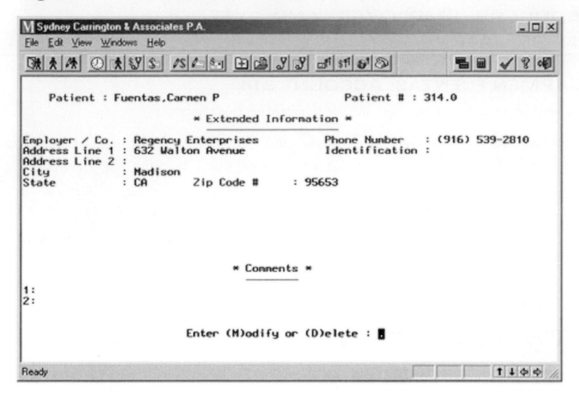

UNIT 4 Editing Prior Entries

EXERCISE 4: CORRECTING A POSTED PROCEDURE AND DIAGNOSIS

MARGARET MORGAN; ACCOUNT 315

When Margaret was seen by the doctor on 04/16/03, the procedure code 99213 was mistakenly entered instead of the code 99214 and the diagnosis, chest pain, was not used for the x-ray.

GOAL(S): Using the information provided above and the encounter form (Figure 4-8, page 64), you will edit the activity to correct the procedure code and add the chest pain diagnosis code to the visit. Enter the chest pain diagnosis with the X-ray Chest PA & Lat procedure. Compare your screen to Figures 4-9 and 4-10.

Figure 4-8 Encounter Form – Morgan

Sydney Carrington & Associates P.A.
34 Sycamore Street   Suite 300
Madison, CA 95653

Date: 04/16/2003   Voucher No.: 3280

Time: 09:00

Patient: Margaret Morgan   Patient No: 315.0
Guarantor: Margaret Morgan   Doctor: 3 - S. Carrington

CPT	DESCRIPTION	FEE		CPT	DESCRIPTION	FEE		CPT	DESCRIPTION	FEE
OFFICE/HOSPITAL CONSULTS				**LABORATORY/RADIOLOGY**				**PROCEDURES/TESTS**		
☐ 99201	Office New:Focused Hx-Exam		☐	81000	Urinalysis		☐	00452	Anesthesia for Rad Surgery	
☐ 99202	Office New:Expanded Hx-Exam		☐	81002	Urinalysis; Pregnancy Test		☐	11100	Skin Biopsy	
☐ 99211	Office Estb:Min/None Hx-Exa		☐	82951	Glucose Tolerance Test		☐	15852	Dressing Change	
☐ 99212	Office Estb:Focused Hx-Exam		☐	84478	Triglycerides		☐	29075	Cast Appl. - Lower Arm	
☐ 99213	Office Estb:Expanded Hx-Exa		☐	84550	Uric Acid: Blood Chemistry		☐	29530	Strapping of Knee	
☒ 99214	Office Estb:Detailed Hx-Exa	$50.00	☐	84830	Ovulation Test		☐	29705	Removal/Revis of Cast w/Exa	
☐ 99215	Office Estb:Comprhn Hx-Exam		☐	85014	Hematocrit		☐	53670	Catheterization Incl. Suppl	
☐ 99221	Hosp. Initial:Comprh Hx-		☐	85031	Hemogram, Complete Blood Wk		☐	57452	Colposcopy	
☐ 99223	Hosp.Ini:Comprh Hx-Exam/Hi		☐	86403	Particle Agglutination Test		☐	57505	ECC	
☐ 99231	Hosp. Subsequent: S-Fwd		☐	86485	Skin Test; Candida		☐	69420	Myringotomy	
☐ 99232	Hosp. Subsequent: Comprhn Hx		☐	86580	TB Intradermal Test		☐	92081	Visual Field Examination	
☐ 99233	Hosp. Subsequent: Ex/Hi		☐	86585	TB Tine Test		☐	92100	Serial Tonometry Exam	
☐ 99238	Hospital Visit Discharge Ex		☐	87070	Culture		☐	92120	Tonography	
☐ 99371	Telephone Consult - Simple		☐	70190	X-Ray; Optic Foramina		☐	92552	Pure Tone Audiometry	
☐ 99372	Telephone Consult - Intermed		☐	70210	X-Ray Sinuses Complete		☐	92567	Tympanometry	
☐ 99373	Telephone Consult - Complex		☐	71010	Radiological Exam Ent Spine		☐	93000	Electrocardiogram	
☐ 90843	Counseling - 25 minutes		☒	71020	X-Ray Chest Pa & Lat	$58.00	☐	93015	Exercise Stress Test (ETT)	
☐ 90844	Counseling - 50 minutes		☐	72050	X-Ray Spine, Cerv (4 views)		☐	93017	ETT Tracing Only	
☐ 90865	Counseling - Special Interview		☐	72090	X-Ray Spine; Scoliosis Ex		☐	93040	Electrocardiogram - Rhythm	
			☐	72110	Spine, lumbosacral; a/p & Lat		☐	96100	Psychological Testing	
IMMUNIZATIONS/INJECTIONS				☐	73030	Shoulder-Comp, min w/ 2vws		☐	99000	Specimen Handling	
☐ 90585	BCG Vaccine		☐	73070	Elbow, anteropost & later vws		☐	99058	Office Emergency Care	
☐ 90659	Influenza Virus Vaccine		☐	73120	X-Ray; Hand, 2 views		☐	99070	Surgical Tray - Misc.	
☐ 90701	Immunization-DTP		☐	73560	X-Ray, Knee, 1 or 2 views		☐	99080	Special Reports of Med Rec	
☐ 90702	DT Vaccine		☐	74022	X-Ray; Abdomen, Complete		☐	99195	Phlebotomy	
☐ 90703	Tetanus Toxoids		☐	75552	Cardiac Magnetic Res Img		☐			
☐ 90732	Pneumococcal Vaccine		☐	76020	X-Ray; Bone Age Studies		☐			
☐ 90746	Hepatitis B Vaccine		☐	76088	Mammary Ductogram Complete		☐			
☐ 90749	Immunization; Unlisted		☐	78465	Myocardial Perfusion Img		☐			

ICD-9 CODE DIAGNOSIS		ICD-9 CODE DIAGNOSIS		ICD-9 CODE DIAGNOSIS	
☐ 009.0	Ill-defined Intestinal Infect	☐ 435.0	Basilar Artery Syndrome	☐ 724.2	Pain: Lower Back
☐ 133.2	Establish Baseline	☐ 440.0	Atherosclerosis	☐ 727.6	Rupture of Achilles Tendon
☐ 174.9	Breast Cancer	☐ 442.81	Carotid Artery	☐ 780.1	Hallucinations
☐ 185.0	Prostate Cancer	☐ 460.0	Common Cold	☐ 780.3	Convulsions
☐ 250	Diabetes Mellitus	☐ 461.9	Acute Sinusitis	☐ 780.5	Sleep Disturbances
☐ 272.4	Hyperlipidemia	☐ 474.0	Tonsillitis	☐ 783.0	Anorexia
☐ 282.5	Anemia - Sickle Trait	☐ 477.9	Hay Fever	☐ 783.1	Abnormal Weight Gain
☐ 282.60	Anemia - Sickle Cell	☐ 487.0	Flu	☐ 783.2	Abnormal Weight Loss
☒ 285.9	Anemia, Unspecified	☐ 496	Chronic Airway Obstruction	☐ 830.6	Dislocated Hip
☐ 300.4	Neurotic Depression	☐ 522	Low Red Blood Count	☐ 830.9	Dislocated Shoulder
☐ 340	Multiple Sclerosis	☐ 524.6	Temporo-Mandibular Jnt Synd	☐ 841.2	Sprained Wrist
☐ 342.9	Hemiplegia - Unspecified	☐ 538.8	Stomach Pain	☐ 842.5	Sprained Ankle
☐ 346.9	Migraine Headache	☐ 553.3	Hiatal Hernia	☐ 891.2	Fractured Tibia
☐ 352.9	Cranial Neuralgia	☐ 564.1	Spastic Colon	☐ 892.0	Fractured Fibula
☐ 354.0	Carpal Tunnel Syndrome	☐ 571.4	Chronic Hepatitis	☐ 919.5	Insect Bite, Nonvenomous
☐ 355.0	Sciatic Nerve Root Lesion	☐ 571.5	Cirrhosis of Liver	☐ 921.1	Contus Eyelid/Perioc Area
☐ 366.9	Cataract	☐ 573.3	Hepatitis	☐ v16.3	Fam. Hist of Breast Cancer
☐ 386.0	Vertigo	☐ 575.2	Obstruction of Gallbladder	☐ v17.4	Fam. Hist of Cardiovasc Dis
☐ 401.1	Essential Hypertension	☐ 648.2	Anemia - Compl. Pregnancy	☐ v20.2	Well Child
☐ 414.9	Ischemic Hearth Disease	☐ 715.90	Osteoarthritis - Unspec	☐ v22.0	Pregnancy - First Normal
☐ 428.0	Congestive Heart Failure	☐ 721.3	Lumbar Osteo/Spondylarthrit	☐ v22.1	Pregnancy - Normal

(786.50)

Previous Balance	Today's Charges	Total Due	Amount Paid	New Balance		Follow Up
0	108.00	108.00	0	108.00	PRN _____ Weeks _____	Months _____ Units _____
					Next Appointment Date:	Time:

I hereby authorize release of any information acquired in the course of
examination or treatment and allow a photocopy of my signature to be used.

_____

Figure 4-9 Corrected Procedure Code

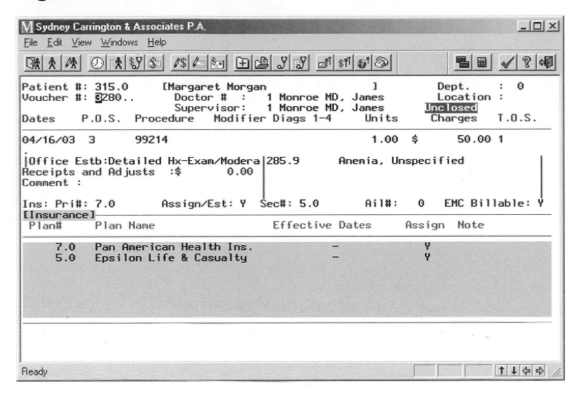

Figure 4-10 Corrected Diagnosis Code

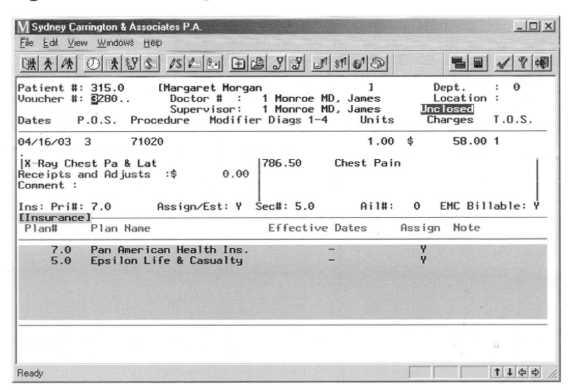

EXERCISE 5: ADDING A DIAGNOSIS TO A POSTED PROCEDURE

SHARON BARKER; ACCOUNT 316

An additional diagnosis code is to be added to Sharon Barker's account for the 04/16/03 visit.

GOAL(S): Using the information provided, you will edit activity to add a second diagnosis code, 724.2 (Pain: Lower Back) to Sharon Barker's account for all three procedures performed. Compare your screen to Figures 4-11, 4-12, and 4-13.

Figure 4-11 Additional diagnosis code - 724.2

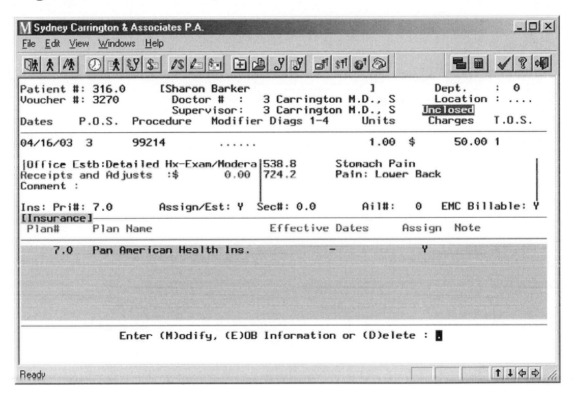

Figure 4-12 Second procedure with added diagnosis code

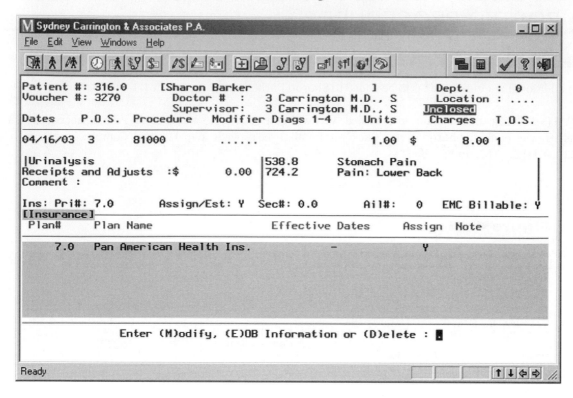

Figure 4-13 Final procedure with diagnosis code 724.2 added

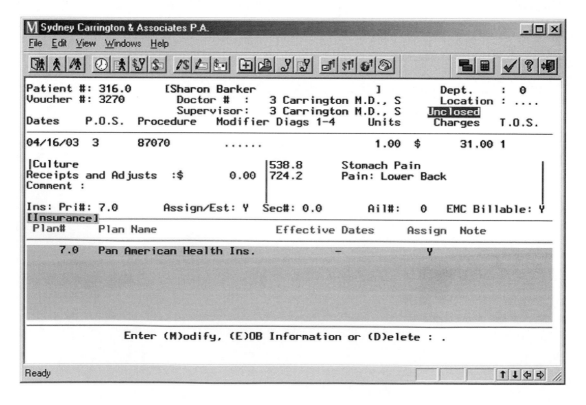

Office Management/ Appointment Scheduling

In the unit exercises that follow, you will use the information provided to schedule individual and multiple appointments, post procedures and schedule follow-up appointments, cancel and reschedule appointments, and print daily list of appointments and hospital rounds report.

EXERCISE 1: SCHEDULE AN APPOINTMENT (TWO WEEKS)

CATHERINE VIAJO

GOAL(S): Schedule an individual appointment in two weeks.

Catherine Viajo calls for an appointment for a general check-up in two weeks. She needs an early morning appointment.

1. Using the information above, schedule Catherine's appointment with Dr. Simpson at 9:30. Compare your screen to Figure 5-1 (page 70).

Figure 5-1 Appointment – Viajo

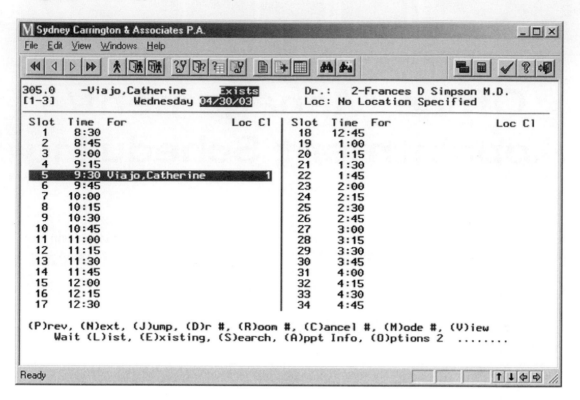

```
M Sydney Carrington & Associates P.A.                              _ □ ×
File  Edit  View  Windows  Help

 ◀◀  ◁  ▷  ▶▶    ⋏ ⬛ ⬛  ⬚⬚ ⬚⬚ ⬚⬚ ⬚⬚   ▤ ⬚ ▦  ⬚⬚ ⬚⬚        ⬚ ▦  ✓ ? ⬚

305.0      -Viajo,Catherine    Exists      Dr.:   2-Frances D Simpson M.D.
[1-3]              Wednesday 04/30/03       Loc: No Location Specified
─────────────────────────────────────────────────────────────────────────
Slot  Time  For              Loc Cl │ Slot  Time   For              Loc Cl
  1   8:30                           │  18   12:45
  2   8:45                           │  19   1:00
  3   9:00                           │  20   1:15
  4   9:15                           │  21   1:30
  5   9:30 Viajo,Catherine        1  │  22   1:45
  6   9:45                           │  23   2:00
  7   10:00                          │  24   2:15
  8   10:15                          │  25   2:30
  9   10:30                          │  26   2:45
 10   10:45                          │  27   3:00
 11   11:00                          │  28   3:15
 12   11:15                          │  29   3:30
 13   11:30                          │  30   3:45
 14   11:45                          │  31   4:00
 15   12:00                          │  32   4:15
 16   12:15                          │  33   4:30
 17   12:30                          │  34   4:45

(P)rev, (N)ext, (J)ump, (D)r #, (R)oom #, (C)ancel #, (M)ode #, (V)iew
      Wait (L)ist, (E)xisting, (S)earch, (A)ppt Info, (O)ptions 2  ........

Ready                                          ⬚  ⬚  ⬚   ↑↓⇦⇨
```

EXERCISE 2: SCHEDULE AN APPOINTMENT (NEXT DAY)

CHRISTINE CUSACK

GOAL(S): Schedule an individual appointment for the next day.

Christine Cusack calls for an appointment for a prenatal exam for tomorrow. She would like an early afternoon appointment.

1. Using the information above, schedule Christine's appointment with Dr. Monroe at 1:00. Compare your screen to Figure 5-2.

Figure 5-2 Appointment – Cusack

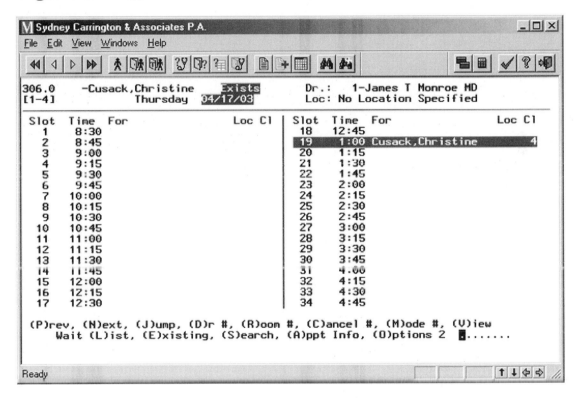

EXERCISE 3: SCHEDULE A MULTI-SLOT APPOINTMENT

JOHN WYATT

GOAL(S): Schedule an appointment with multiple slots in three weeks.

John Wyatt calls for an appointment for a personal consult in three weeks. He needs a late afternoon appointment.

1. Using the information above, schedule John's appointment with Dr. Monroe at 4:00 for 30 minutes. Compare your screen to Figure 5-3.

Figure 5-3 Appointment – Wyatt

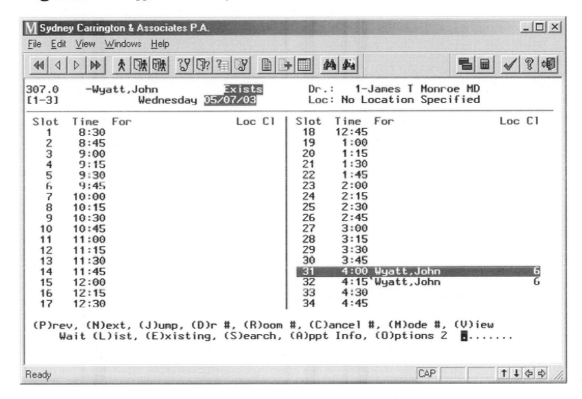

EXERCISE 4: SCHEDULE ANOTHER MULTI-SLOT APPOINTMENT

LINDA FROST

GOAL(S): Schedule an appointment with multiple slots for Monday, 04/21/03.

Linda Frost needs to have an x-ray done on her wrist. She cannot come into the office until Monday. She would like a morning appointment.

1. Using the information above, schedule Linda's appointment with Dr. Carrington at 10:00 for 30 minutes. Compare your screen to Figure 5-4.

Figure 5-4   Appointment – Frost

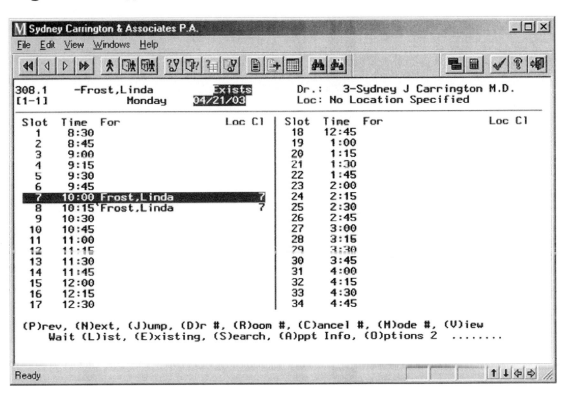

EXERCISE 5: SCHEDULE AN APPOINTMENT CONFLICT

JUAN PEREZ

GOAL(S): Schedule an appointment for Monday, 04/21/03, creating an appointment conflict.

Juan Perez calls to schedule a general check-up at 10:15 on Monday, 04/21/03. He would like to see Dr. Carrington.

1. Using the information above, schedule Juan's appointment, accepting the conflict. Compare your screen to Figure 5-5.

Figure 5-5 Appointment Conflict

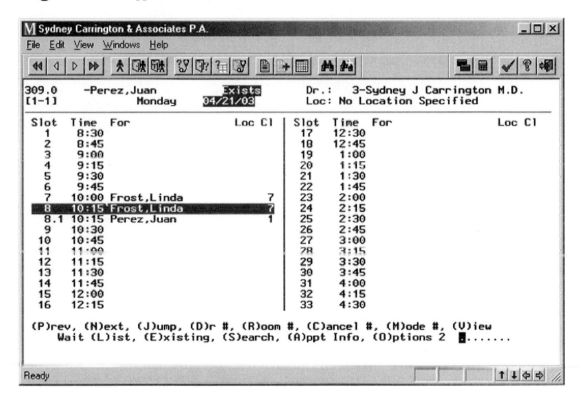

EXERCISE 6: SCHEDULE A DIFFERENT DOCTOR

MATTHEW NOONAN

GOAL(S): Schedule an appointment with a different doctor.

Matthew Noonan needs an appointment for an annual check-up in two weeks and he would like to see Dr. Monroe.

1. Key '?NOONAN' to retrieve Matthew Noonan by name.

2. Using the information above, schedule Matthew's appointment with Dr. Monroe at 3:30. Compare your screen to Figure 5-6.

Figure 5-6 Appointment with Dr. Monroe

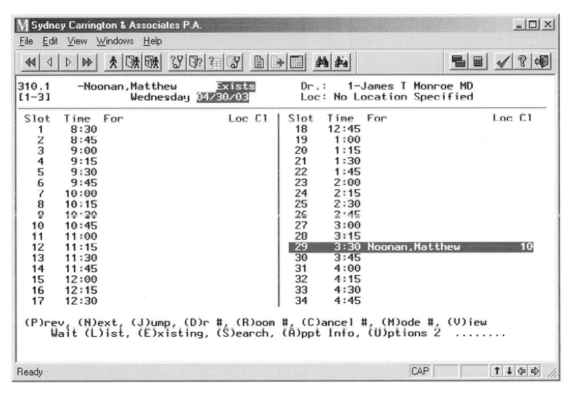

EXERCISE 7: DAILY LIST OF APPOINTMENTS

GOAL(S): Prepare an Appointments Detail Report by doctor.

1. Print an Appointments Detail Report by doctor, with remarks. Select only doctors 1-3 to print. Select the starting date as 04/16/03 and ending date as 05/15/03. Enter for all locations. Give your reports to your instructor.

EXERCISE 8: RESCHEDULE AN APPOINTMENT

CHRISTOPHER SALVANI

GOAL(S): Reschedule an appointment.

Christopher Salvani's appointment for a general check-up on April 24 at 2:30 with Dr. Simpson needs to be rescheduled for April 30.

1. Reschedule Christopher's general check-up appointment for 1:45 on April 30 with Dr. Simpson. Use CALLED as the reason code. Compare your screen to Figure 5-7.

Figure 5-7   Rescheduled Appointment

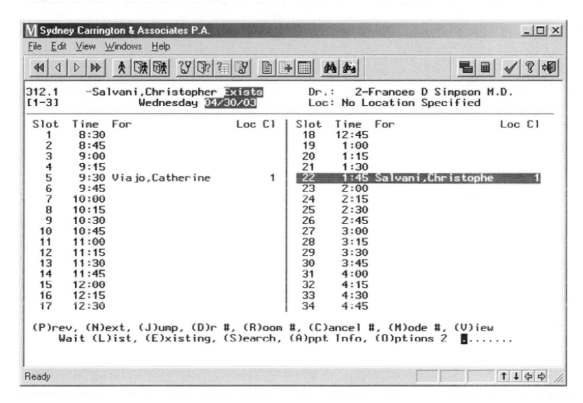

EXERCISE 9: RESCHEDULE WITH A DIFFERENT DOCTOR

DAVID FUENTAS

GOAL(S): Correct a scheduling error by rescheduling an appointment with a different doctor.

David Fuentas's personal consult appointment on April 18 at 11:30 was mistakenly entered on Dr. Carrington's schedule.

1. Using the information above, reschedule David's appointment for Dr. Monroe at 11:30 on April 18. Use ERROR for the reason code. Compare your screen to Figure 5-8.

Figure 5-8 Rescheduled – Fuentas

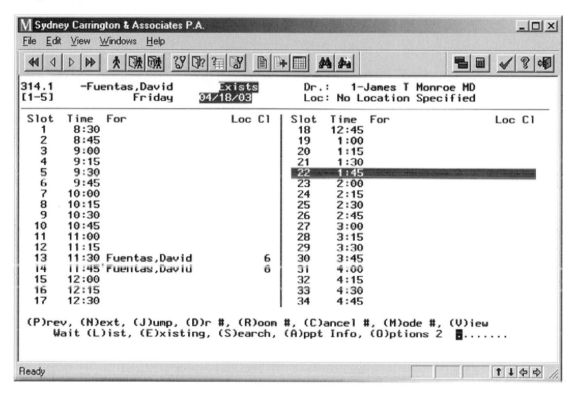

EXERCISE 10: CANCELING AN APPOINTMENT

MARGARET MORGAN

GOAL(S): Cancel an appointment.

Margaret Morgan called to cancel a recheck appointment that is scheduled for April 17 with Dr. Carrington at 2:00.

  1. Retrieve Margaret's account and cancel her appointment. Use CALL24 as the cancel code.

EXERCISE 11: POSTING PROCEDURES AND FOLLOW-UP APPOINTMENT

SONIA LOPEZ

GOAL(S): Post procedures and schedule an appointment.

1. Post the procedures from Sonia's encounter form using the information in Figure 5-9. Compare your screen to Figure 5-10.

Figure 5-9 Encounter Form – Lopez

<table>
<tr><td colspan="3" align="center">

Sydney Carrington & Associates P.A.
34 Sycamore Street   Suite 300
Madison, CA 95653
</td></tr>
</table>

Date: 04/16/2003   Voucher No.: 5001

Time:

Patient: Sonia Lopez   Patient No: 317.0
Guarantor: Doctor: 2 - F. Simpson

CPT	DESCRIPTION	FEE	CPT	DESCRIPTION	FEE	CPT	DESCRIPTION	FEE
OFFICE/HOSPITAL CONSULTS			**LABORATORY/RADIOLOGY**			**PROCEDURES/TESTS**		
☐ 99201	Office New:Focused Hx-Exam		☐ 81000	Urinalysis		☐ 00452	Anesthesia for Rad Surgery	
☐ 99202	Office New:Expanded Hx-Exam		☐ 81002	Urinalysis; Pregnancy Test		☐ 11100	Skin Biopsy	
☐ 99211	Office Estb:Min/None Hx-Exa		☐ 82951	Glucose Tolerance Test		☐ 15852	Dressing Change	
☐ 99212	Office Estb:Focused Hx-Exam		☐ 84478	Triglycerides		☐ 29075	Cast Appl. - Lower Arm	
☒ 99213	Office Estb:Expanded Hx Exa		☐ 84550	Uric Acid: Blood Chemistry		☐ 29530	Strapping of Knee	
☐ 99214	Office Estb:Detailed Hx-Exa		☐ 84830	Ovulation Test		☐ 29705	Removal/Revis of Cast w/Exa	
☐ 99215	Office Estb:Comprhn Hx Exam		☐ 85014	Hematocrit		☐ 53670	Catheterization Incl. Suppl	
☐ 99221	Hosp. Initial:Comprh Hx-		☒ 85031	Hemogram, Complete Blood Wk		☐ 57452	Colposcopy	
☐ 99223	Hosp.Ini.Comprh Hx-Exam/Hi		☐ 00403	Particle Agglutination Test		☐ 57505	ECG	
☐ 99231	Hosp. Subsequent: S-Fwd		☐ 86485	Skin Test; Candida		☐ 69420	Myringotomy	
☐ 99232	Hosp. Subsequent: Comprhn Hx		☐ 86580	TB Intradermal Test		☐ 92081	Visual Field Examination	
☐ 99233	Hosp. Subsequent: Ex/Hi		☐ 86585	TB Tine Test		☐ 92100	Serial Tonometry Exam	
☐ 99238	Hospital Visit Discharge Ex		☐ 87070	Culture		☐ 92120	Tonography	
☐ 99371	Telephone Consult - Simple		☐ 70190	X-Ray; Optic Foramina		☐ 92552	Pure Tone Audiometry	
☐ 99372	Telephone Consult - Intermed		☐ 70210	X-Ray Sinuses Complete		☐ 92567	Tympanometry	
☐ 99373	Telephone Consult - Complex		☐ 71010	Radiological Exam Ent Spine		☐ 93000	Electrocardiogram	
☐ 90843	Counseling - 25 minutes		☐ 71020	X-Ray Chest Pa & Lat		☐ 93015	Exercise Stress Test (ETT)	
☐ 90844	Counseling - 50 minutes		☐ 72050	X-Ray Spine, Cerv (4 views)		☐ 93017	ETT Tracing Only	
☐ 90865	Counseling - Special Interview		☐ 72090	X-Ray Spine; Scoliosis Ex		☐ 93040	Electrocardiogram - Rhythm	
			☐ 72110	Spine, lumbosacral; a/p & Lat		☐ 96100	Psychological Testing	
IMMUNIZATIONS/INJECTIONS			☐ 73030	Shoulder-Comp, min w/ 2vws		☐ 99000	Specimen Handling	
☐ 90585	BCG Vaccine		☐ 73070	Elbow, anteropost & later vws		☐ 99058	Office Emergency Care	
☐ 90659	Influenza Virus Vaccine		☐ 73120	X-Ray; Hand, 2 views		☐ 99070	Surgical Tray - Misc.	
☐ 90701	Immunization-DTP		☐ 73560	X-Ray, Knee, 1 or 2 views		☐ 99080	Special Reports of Med Rec	
☐ 90702	DT Vaccine		☐ 74022	X-Ray; Abdomen, Complete		☐ 99195	Phlebotomy	
☐ 90703	Tetanus Toxoids		☐ 75552	Cardiac Magnetic Res Img		☐	_____	
☐ 90732	Pneumococcal Vaccine		☐ 76020	X-Ray; Bone Age Studies		☐	_____	
☐ 90746	Hepatitis B Vaccine		☐ 76088	Mammary Ductogram Complete		☐	_____	
☐ 90749	Immunization; Unlisted		☐ 78465	Myocardial Perfusion Img				

CPT	ICD-9 CODE DIAGNOSIS		CPT	ICD-9 CODE DIAGNOSIS		CPT	ICD-9 CODE DIAGNOSIS	
☐ 009.0	Ill-defined Intestinal Infect		☐ 435.0	Basilar Artery Syndrome		☐ 724.2	Pain: Lower Back	
☐ 100.0	Establish Baseline		☐ 440.0	Atherosclerosis		☐ 727.6	Rupture of Achilles Tendon	
☐ 174.9	Breast Cancer		☐ 442.81	Carotid Artery		☐ 780.1	Hallucinations	
☐ 185.0	Prostate Cancer		☐ 460.0	Common Cold		☐ 780.3	Convulsions	
☐ 250	Diabetes Mellitus		☐ 461.9	Acute Sinusitis		☐ 780.5	Sleep Disturbances	
☐ 272.4	Hyperlipidemia		☐ 474.0	Tonsillitis		☐ 783.0	Anorexia	
☐ 282.5	Anemia - Sickle Trait		☐ 477.9	Hay Fever		☐ 783.1	Abnormal Weight Gain	
☐ 282.60	Anemia - Sickle Cell		☐ 487.0	Flu		☒ 783.2	Abnormal Weight Loss	
☐ 285.9	Anemia, Unspecified		☐ 496	Chronic Airway Obstruction		☐ 830.6	Dislocated Hip	
☐ 300.4	Neurotic Depression		☐ 522	Low Red Blood Count		☐ 830.9	Dislocated Shoulder	
☐ 340	Multiple Sclerosis		☐ 524.6	Temporo-Mandibular Jnt Synd		☐ 841.2	Sprained Wrist	
☐ 342.9	Hemiplegia - Unspecified		☐ 538.8	Stomach Pain		☐ 842.5	Sprained Ankle	
☐ 346.9	Migraine Headache		☐ 553.3	Hiatal Hernia		☐ 891.2	Fractured Tibia	
☐ 352.9	Cranial Neuralgia		☐ 564.1	Spastic Colon		☐ 892.0	Fractured Fibula	
☐ 354.0	Carpal Tunnel Syndrome		☐ 571.4	Chronic Hepatitis		☐ 919.5	Insect Bite, Nonvenomous	
☐ 355.0	Sciatic Nerve Root Lesion		☐ 571.5	Cirrhosis of Liver		☐ 921.1	Contus Eyelid/Perioc Area	
☐ 366.9	Cataract		☐ 573.3	Hepatitis		☐ v16.3	Fam. Hist of Breast Cancer	
☐ 386.0	Vertigo		☐ 575.2	Obstruction of Gallbladder		☐ v17.4	Fam. Hist of Cardiovasc Dis	
☐ 401.1	Essential Hypertension		☐ 648.2	Anemia - Compl. Pregnancy		☐ v20.2	Well Child	
☐ 414.9	Ischemic Hearth Disease		☐ 715.90	Osteoarthritis - Unspec		☐ v22.0	Pregnancy - First Normal	
☐ 428.0	Congestive Heart Failure		☐ 721.3	Lumbar Osteo/Spondylarthrit		☐ v22.1	Pregnancy - Normal	

Previous Balance	Today's Charges	Total Due	Amount Paid	New Balance		Follow Up				
						PRN _____ Weeks _____	Months _____	Units _____		
_____	_____	_____	_____	_____		Next Appointment Date: Apr. 23 Time: 10:45 Recheck				

I hereby authorize release of any information acquired in the course of examination or treatment and allow a photocopy of my signature to be used.

_____

2. Schedule Sonia's next appointment as indicated on her encounter form. Compare your screen to Figure 5-11.

Figure 5-10 Two Procedures Posted

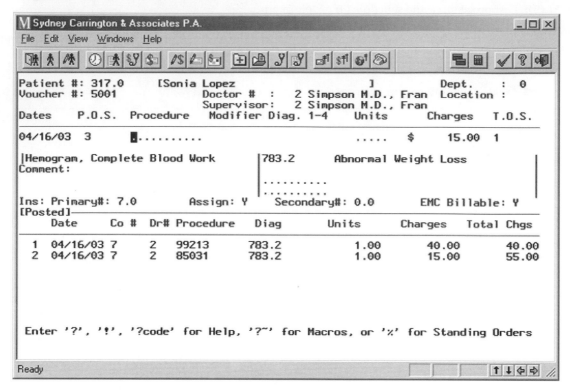

Figure 5-11 Follow-up Appointment – Lopez

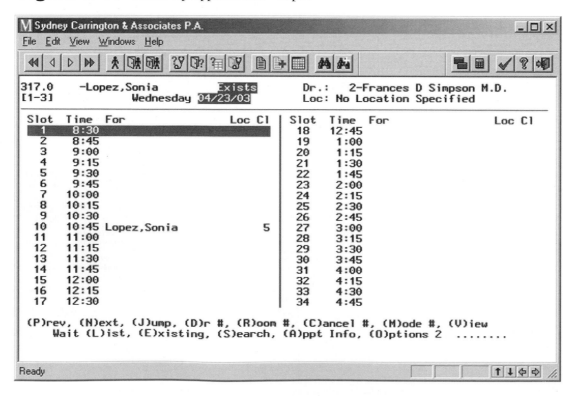

EXERCISE 12: POST PROCEDURES AND MULTI-SLOT FOLLOW-UP APPOINTMENT

GARY BRINKMAN

GOAL(S): Post procedures and schedule an appointment for a multiple slot.

Figure 5-12 Encounter Form – Brinkman

Sydney Carrington & Associates P.A.
34 Sycamore Street   Suite 300
Madison, CA 95653

Date: 04/16/2003

Voucher No.: 5002

Time:

Patient: Gary Brinkman
Guarantor:

Patient No: 318.0
Doctor: 1 - J. Monroe

	CPT	DESCRIPTION	FEE		CPT	DESCRIPTION	FEE		CPT	DESCRIPTION	FEE
OFFICE/HOSPITAL CONSULTS				**LABORATORY/RADIOLOGY**				**PROCEDURES/TESTS**			
☐	00201	Office New:Focused Hx-Exam		☒	81000	Urinalysis		☐	00452	Anesthesia for Rad Surgery	
☐	99202	Office New:Expanded Hx-Exam		☐	81002	Urinalysis; Pregnancy Test		☐	11100	Skin Biopsy	
☐	99211	Office Estb:Min/None Hx-Exa		☒	82951	Glucose Tolerance Test		☐	15852	Dressing Change	
☐	99212	Office Estb:Focused Hx-Exam		☐	84478	Triglycerides		☐	29075	Cast Appl. - Lower Arm	
☐	99213	Office Estb:Expanded Hx-Exa		☐	84550	Uric Acid: Blood Chemistry		☐	29530	Strapping of Knee	
☒	99214	Office Estb:Detailed Hx-Exa		☐	84830	Ovulation Test		☐	29705	Removal/Revis of Cast w/Exa	
☐	99215	Office Estb:Comprhn Hx-Exam		☐	85014	Hematocrit		☐	53670	Catheterization Incl. Suppl	
☐	99221	Hosp. Initial:Comprh Hx-		☐	85031	Hemogram, Complete Blood Wk		☐	57452	Colposcopy	
☐	99223	Hosp.Ini:Comprh Hx-Exam/Hi		☐	86403	Particle Agglutination Test		☐	57505	ECC	
☐	99231	Hosp. Subsequent: S-Fwd		☐	86485	Skin Test; Candida		☐	69420	Myringotomy	
☐	99232	Hosp. Subsequent: Comprhn Hx		☐	86580	TB Intradermal Test		☐	92081	Visual Field Examination	
☐	99233	Hosp. Subsequent. Ex/Hi		☐	86585	TB Tine Test		☐	92100	Serial Tonometry Exam	
☐	99238	Hospital Visit Discharge Ex		☐	87070	Culture		☐	92120	Tonography	
☐	99371	Telephone Consult - Simple		☐	70190	X-Ray; Optic Foramina		☐	92552	Pure Tone Audiometry	
☐	99372	Telephone Consult - Intermed		☐	70210	X-Ray Sinuses Complete		☐	92567	Tympanometry	
☐	99373	Telephone Consult - Complex		☐	71010	Radiological Exam Ent Spine		☐	93000	Electrocardiogram	
☐	90843	Counseling - 25 minutes		☐	71020	X-Ray Chest Pa & Lat		☐	93015	Exercise Stress Test (ETT)	
☐	90844	Counseling - 50 minutes		☐	72050	X-Ray Spine, Cerv (4 views)		☐	93017	ETT Tracing Only	
☐	90865	Counseling - Special Interview		☐	72090	X-Ray Spine; Scoliosis Ex		☐	93040	Electrocardiogram - Rhythm	
				☐	72110	Spine, lumbosacral; a/p & Lat		☐	96100	Psychological Testing	
IMMUNIZATIONS/INJECTIONS				☐	73030	Shoulder-Comp, min w/ 2vws		☐	99000	Specimen Handling	
☐	90585	BCG Vaccine		☐	73070	Elbow, anteropost & later vws		☐	99058	Office Emergency Care	
☐	90659	Influenza Virus Vaccine		☐	73120	X-Ray; Hand, 2 views		☐	99070	Surgical Tray - Misc.	
☐	90701	Immunization-DTP		☐	73560	X-Ray, Knee, 1 or 2 views		☐	99080	Special Reports of Med Rec	
☐	90702	DT Vaccine		☐	74022	X-Ray; Abdomen, Complete		☐	99195	Phlebotomy	
☐	90703	Tetanus Toxoids		☐	75552	Cardiac Magnetic Res Img		☐			
☐	90732	Pneumococcal Vaccine		☐	76020	X-Ray; Bone Age Studies		☐			
☐	90746	Hepatitis B Vaccine		☐	76088	Mammary Ductogram Complete		☐			
☐	90749	Immunization; Unlisted		☐	78465	Myocardial Perfusion Img		☐			

	ICD-9 CODE DIAGNOSIS			ICD-9 CODE DIAGNOSIS			ICD-9 CODE DIAGNOSIS	
☐	009.0	Ill-defined Intestinal Infect	☐	435.0	Basilar Artery Syndrome	☐	724.2	Pain: Lower Back
☐	133.2	Establish Baseline	☐	440.0	Atherosclerosis	☐	727.6	Rupture of Achilles Tendon
☐	174.9	Breast Cancer	☐	442.81	Carotid Artery	☐	780.1	Hallucinations
☐	185.0	Prostate Cancer	☐	460.0	Common Cold	☐	780.3	Convulsions
☒	250	Diabetes Mellitus	☐	461.9	Acute Sinusitis	☐	780.5	Sleep Disturbances
☐	272.4	Hyperlipidemia	☐	474.0	Tonsillitis	☐	783.0	Anorexia
☐	282.5	Anemia - Sickle Trait	☐	477.9	Hay Fever	☐	783.1	Abnormal Weight Gain
☐	282.60	Anemia - Sickle Cell	☐	487.0	Flu	☐	783.2	Abnormal Weight Loss
☐	285.9	Anemia, Unspecified	☐	496	Chronic Airway Obstruction	☐	830.6	Dislocated Hip
☐	300.4	Neurotic Depression	☐	522	Low Red Blood Count	☐	830.9	Dislocated Shoulder
☐	340	Multiple Sclerosis	☐	524.6	Temporo-Mandibular Jnt Synd	☐	841.2	Sprained Wrist
☐	342.9	Hemiplegia - Unspecified	☐	538.8	Stomach Pain	☐	842.5	Sprained Ankle
☐	346.9	Migraine Headache	☐	553.3	Hiatal Hernia	☐	891.2	Fractured Tibia
☐	352.9	Cranial Neuralgia	☐	564.1	Spastic Colon	☐	892.0	Fractured Fibula
☐	354.0	Carpal Tunnel Syndrome	☐	571.4	Chronic Hepatitis	☐	919.5	Insect Bite, Nonvenomous
☐	355.0	Sciatic Nerve Root Lesion	☐	571.5	Cirrhosis of Liver	☐	921.1	Contus Eyelid/Perioc Area
☐	366.9	Cataract	☐	573.3	Hepatitis	☐	v16.3	Fam. Hist of Breast Cancer
☐	386.0	Vertigo	☐	575.2	Obstruction of Gallbladder	☐	v17.4	Fam. Hist of Cardiovasc Dis
☐	401.1	Essential Hypertension	☐	648.2	Anemia - Compl. Pregnancy	☐	v20.2	Well Child
☐	414.9	Ischemic Hearth Disease	☐	715.90	Osteoarthritis - Unspec	☐	v22.0	Pregnancy - First Normal
☐	428.0	Congestive Heart Failure	☐	721.3	Lumbar Osteo/Spondylarthrit	☐	v22.1	Pregnancy - Normal

Previous Balance	Today's Charges	Total Due	Amount Paid	New Balance

Follow Up

PRN _____ Weeks _____ Months _____ Units _____

Next Appointment Date: Apr. 18   Time: 8:15   Personal consult; 30 minutes

I hereby authorize release of any information acquired in the course of examination or treatment and allow a photocopy of my signature to be used.

_____

1. Post three procedures from Gary's encounter form. Compare your screen to Figure 5-13.

2. Schedule Gary's next appointment as indicated on his encounter form. Compare your screen to Figure 5-14.

Figure 5-13 Three Procedures Posted – Brinkman

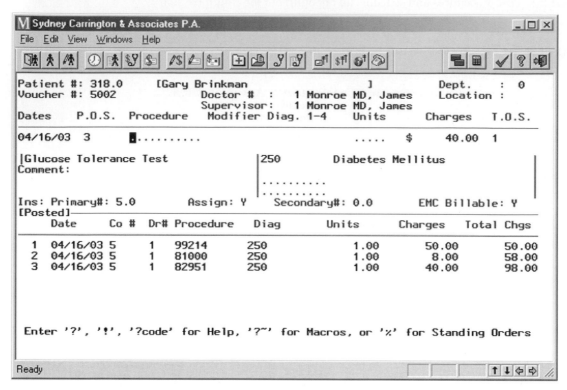

Figure 5-14 Return Appointment – Brinkman

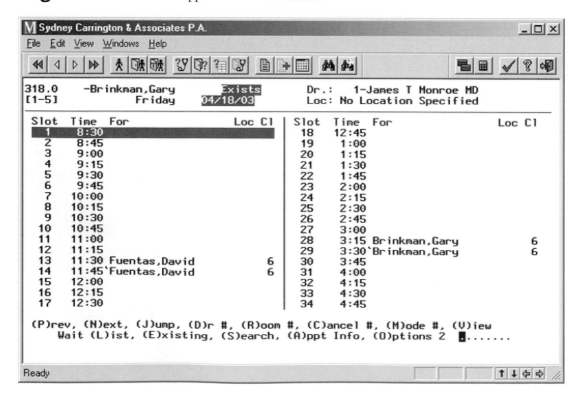

EXERCISE 13: CANCEL AN APPOINTMENT AND ADD HOSPITAL ROUNDS

GARY BRINKMAN

GOAL(S): In this exercise you will cancel an existing appointment, add a patient to a hospital rounds report, and print the report.

Gary Brinkman calls the office later the same day, following his last appointment (Exercise 12). Dr. Monroe is going to admit Gary Brinkman to Jefferson Memorial Hospital due to his diabetic condition. He is expected to be in the hospital for three days. Use the information provided to create the report.

1. Cancel Gary's existing appointment on April 18.

2. Add Gary to hospital rounds to have this entry appear on Dr. Monroe's rounds report.

3. Gary's hospital ID # is 157239630.

4. Gary's admission is urgent. Compare your screen to Figure 5-15.

5. Print a hospital rounds report sorted by doctor, including tomorrow's admissions, for all doctors and facilities. Give your report to your instructor.

Figure 5-15 Hospital Admission

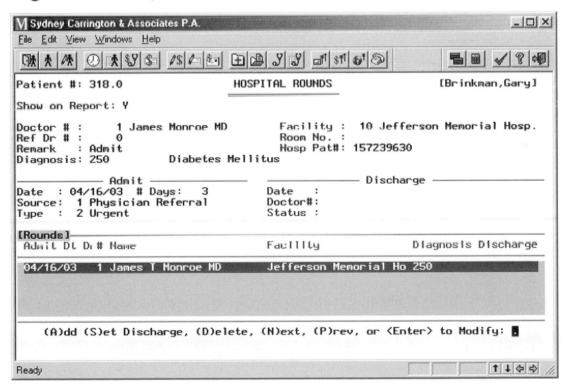

EXERCISE 14: POST PROCEDURE CODES FOR HOSPITAL VISITS

GOAL(S): In this exercise you will need to use the procedure code help window to locate codes.

Dr. Monroe has discharged Gary Brinkman from Jefferson Memorial Hospital after his four-day stay. Using the Hospital Rounds report (Figure 5-16) and the information provided below, post the charges to his account.

Figure 5-16 Hospital Rounds Report

```
04/16/03                        HOSPITAL ROUNDS REPORT BY SERVICE FACILITY              Page    1
                                    Sydney Carrington & Associates P.A.
                                         (1)James T Monroe MD
                                            All Facilities


 Patient                        Pat #   DOB        Admit Info                Referring Dr.      Remark
==============================================================================================
------------------------------------
Jefferson Memorial Hosp.   (10)
------------------------------------
  Brinkman,Gary                 318.0   11/04/1960  Date  : 04/16/03  Days: 3                    Admit
                                                    Source: Physician Referral  Phone:
    Room:               Hosp ID: 157239630          Type  : Urgent             Notes:
    Diag: 250           Diabetes Mellitus
                                                    ------------------------

          Discharge to home  04/19/03
```

Become familiar with the hospital rounds report and answer the following questions before attempting the data entry:

1. What is the date of admission for Gary Brinkman?

2. What is the date of discharge for Gary Brinkman?

3. Which doctor cared for Gary Brinkman during his hospital stay?

Gary Brinkman's hospitalization charges will include:

04/16/03	One Procedure: Admission History and Comprehensive Physical Exam (Hospital Initial: Comprh Hx-Exam/Hi)
04/17/03, 04/18/03	Two Procedures: Hospital Visit Expanded (Hosp. Subsequent: Comprh Hx-Exam/Mod)
04/19/03	One Procedure: Hospital Discharge Exam (Hospital Visit Discharge Exam)

When you have posted the hospital visits listed above, compare your screen to Figure 5-17.

Figure 5-17   Posted – Three Hospital Visits

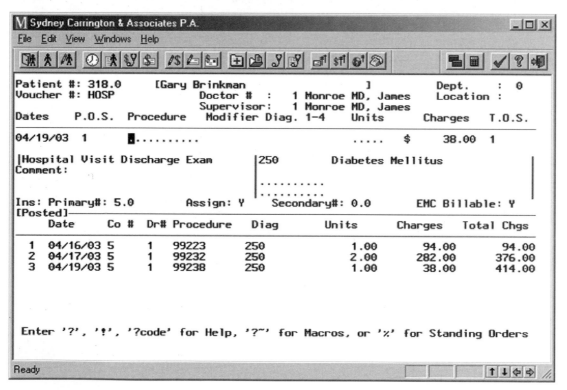

Practice Management

In the unit exercises that follow, you will post procedures, post patient payments, post negative adjustments, transfer payment responsibility, use automatic crediting, and post insurance payments.

EXERCISE 1: POST PROCEDURES AND PATIENT PAYMENT

WAYNE MILES; ACCOUNT 319

GOAL(S): In this exercise you will post procedures and payments from the Procedure Entry screen for Wayne Miles, who will pay in full for the visit.

1. Before posting your entry, study the encounter form in Figure 6-1 (page 98). Answer the following questions:

   a. How many procedures were performed? _____

   b. What is the diagnosis? _____

   c. What is the total charge for this visit? _____

2. Based on the information found on the encounter form, post the charges for Wayne Miles. When you have correctly posted all three procedures, compare your screen to Figure 6-2.

3. Wayne Miles provides a check for the full amount of the visit. See Figure 6-3. Apply the check for $123 to his account. Compare your screen to Figure 6-4.

Figure 6-1 Encounter Form – Miles

Sydney Carrington & Associates P.A.
34 Sycamore Street   Suite 300
Madison, CA 95653

Date: 04/16/2003

Time:

Patient: Wayne Miles
Guarantor:

Voucher No.: 1163

Patient No: 319.0
Doctor: 2 - F. Simpson

	CPT	DESCRIPTION	FEE
	OFFICE/HOSPITAL CONSULTS		
☐	99201	Office New:Focused Hx-Exam	
☐	99202	Office New:Expanded Hx-Exam	
☐	99211	Office Estb:Min/None Hx-Exa	
☐	99212	Office Estb:Focused Hx-Exam	
☐	99213	Office Estb:Expanded Hx-Exa	
☒	99214	Office Estb:Detailed Hx-Exa	$50
☐	99215	Office Estb:Comprhn Hx-Exam	
☐	99221	Hosp. Initial:Comprh Hx-	
☐	99223	Hosp.Ini:Comprh Hx-Exam/Hi	
☐	99231	Hosp. Subsequent: S-Fwd	
☐	99232	Hosp. Subsequent: Comprhn Hx	
☐	99233	Hosp. Subsequent: Ex/Hi	
☐	99238	Hospital Visit Discharge Ex	
☐	99371	Telephone Consult - Simple	
☐	99372	Telephone Consult - Intermed	
☐	99373	Telephone Consult - Complex	
☐	90843	Counseling - 25 minutes	
☐	90844	Counseling - 50 minutes	
☐	90865	Counseling - Special Interview	
	IMMUNIZATIONS/INJECTIONS		
☐	90585	BCG Vaccine	
☐	90659	Influenza Virus Vaccine	
☐	90701	Immunization-DTP	
☐	90702	DT Vaccine	
☐	90703	Tetanus Toxoids	
☐	90732	Pneumococcal Vaccine	
☐	90746	Hepatitis B Vaccine	
☐	90749	Immunization; Unlisted	

	CPT	DESCRIPTION	FEE
	LABORATORY/RADIOLOGY		
☐	81000	Urinalysis	
☐	81002	Urinalysis; Pregnancy Test	
☐	82951	Glucose Tolerance Test	
☐	84478	Triglycerides	
☐	84550	Uric Acid: Blood Chemistry	
☐	84830	Ovulation Test	
☐	85014	Hematocrit	
☒	85031	Hemogram, Complete Blood Wk	$15
☐	86403	Particle Agglutination Test	
☐	86485	Skin Test; Candida	
☐	86580	TB Intradermal Test	
☐	86585	TB Tine Test	
☐	87070	Culture	
☐	70190	X-Ray; Optic Foramina	
☐	70210	X-Ray Sinuses Complete	
☐	71010	Radiological Exam Ent Spine	
☒	71020	X-Ray Chest Pa & Lat	$58
☐	72050	X-Ray Spine, Cerv (4 views)	
☐	72090	X-Ray Spine; Scoliosis Ex	
☐	72110	Spine, lumbosacral; a/p & Lat	
☐	73030	Shoulder-Comp, min w/ 2vws	
☐	73070	Elbow, anteropost & later vws	
☐	73120	X-Ray; Hand, 2 views	
☐	73560	X-Ray, Knee, 1 or 2 views	
☐	74022	X-Ray; Abdomen, Complete	
☐	75552	Cardiac Magnetic Res Img	
☐	76020	X-Ray; Bone Age Studies	
☐	76088	Mammary Ductogram Complete	
☐	78465	Myocardial Perfusion Img	

	CPT	DESCRIPTION	FEE
	PROCEDURES/TESTS		
☐	00452	Anesthesia for Rad Surgery	
☐	11100	Skin Biopsy	
☐	15852	Dressing Change	
☐	29075	Cast Appl. - Lower Arm	
☐	29530	Strapping of Knee	
☐	29705	Removal/Revis of Cast w/Exa	
☐	53670	Catheterization Incl. Suppl	
☐	57452	Colposcopy	
☐	57505	ECC	
☐	69420	Myringotomy	
☐	92081	Visual Field Examination	
☐	92100	Serial Tonometry Exam	
☐	92120	Tonography	
☐	92552	Pure Tone Audiometry	
☐	92567	Tympanometry	
☐	93000	Electrocardiogram	
☐	93015	Exercise Stress Test (ETT)	
☐	93017	ETT Tracing Only	
☐	93040	Electrocardiogram - Rhythm	
☐	96100	Psychological Testing	
☐	99000	Specimen Handling	
☐	99058	Office Emergency Care	
☐	99070	Surgical Tray - Misc.	
☐	99080	Special Reports of Med Rec	
☐	99195	Phlebotomy	
☐			
☐			
☐			

	ICD-9 CODE DIAGNOSIS	
☐	009.0	Ill-defined Intestinal Infect
☐	133.2	Establish Baseline
☐	174.9	Breast Cancer
☐	185.0	Prostate Cancer
☐	250	Diabetes Mellitus
☐	272.4	Hyperlipidemia
☐	282.5	Anemia - Sickle Trait
☐	282.60	Anemia - Sickle Cell
☐	285.9	Anemia, Unspecified
☐	300.4	Neurotic Depression
☐	340	Multiple Sclerosis
☐	342.9	Hemiplegia - Unspecified
☐	346.9	Migraine Headache
☐	352.9	Cranial Neuralgia
☐	354.0	Carpal Tunnel Syndrome
☐	355.0	Sciatic Nerve Root Lesion
☐	366.9	Cataract
☐	386.0	Vertigo
☐	401.1	Essential Hypertension
☐	414.9	Ischemic Hearth Disease
☐	428.0	Congestive Heart Failure

	ICD-9 CODE DIAGNOSIS	
☐	435.0	Basilar Artery Syndrome
☐	440.0	Atherosclerosis
☐	442.81	Carotid Artery
☐	460.0	Common Cold
☐	461.9	Acute Sinusitis
☐	474.0	Tonsillitis
☐	477.9	Hay Fever
☐	487.0	Flu
☐	496	Chronic Airway Obstruction
☐	522	Low Red Blood Count
☐	524.6	Temporo-Mandibular Jnt Synd
☐	538.8	Stomach Pain
☐	553.3	Hiatal Hernia
☐	564.1	Spastic Colon
☐	571.4	Chronic Hepatitis
☐	571.5	Cirrhosis of Liver
☐	573.3	Hepatitis
☐	575.2	Obstruction of Gallbladder
☐	648.2	Anemia - Compl. Pregnancy
☐	715.90	Osteoarthritis - Unspec
☐	721.3	Lumbar Osteo/Spondylarthrit

	ICD-9 CODE DIAGNOSIS	
☐	724.2	Pain: Lower Back
☐	727.6	Rupture of Achilles Tendon
☐	780.1	Hallucinations
☐	780.3	Convulsions
☐	780.5	Sleep Disturbances
☐	783.0	Anorexia
☐	783.1	Abnormal Weight Gain
☐	783.2	Abnormal Weight Loss
☐	830.6	Dislocated Hip
☐	830.9	Dislocated Shoulder
☐	841.2	Sprained Wrist
☐	842.5	Sprained Ankle
☐	891.2	Fractured Tibia
☐	892.0	Fractured Fibula
☐	919.5	Insect Bite, Nonvenomous
☐	921.1	Contus Eyelid/Perioc Area
☐	v16.3	Fam. Hist of Breast Cancer
☐	v17.4	Fam. Hist of Cardiovasc Dis
☐	v20.2	Well Child
☐	v22.0	Pregnancy - First Normal
☐	v22.1	Pregnancy - Normal
X	480.0	Viral Pneumonia

Previous Balance	Today's Charges	Total Due	Amount Paid	New Balance
_____	_____	_____	$123 check #1624	

Follow Up

PRN _____ Weeks _____ Months _____ Units _____

Next Appointment Date: Time:

I hereby authorize release of any information acquired in the course of
examination or treatment and allow a photocopy of my signature to be used.

_____

Figure 6-2 Three Procedures Posted – Miles

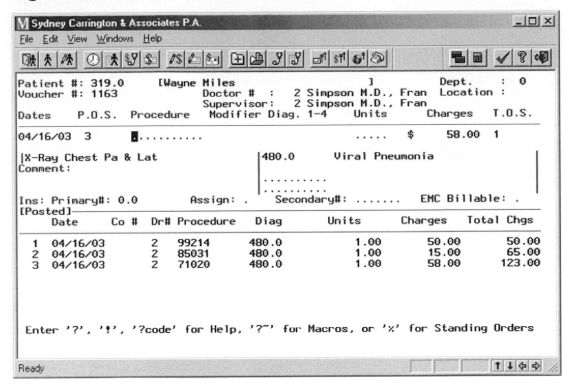

```
M  Sydney Carrington & Associates P.A.                                    _ □ ×
File  Edit  View  Windows  Help

┌──┬──┬──┬──┬──┬──┬──┬──┬──┬──┬──┬──┬──┬──┬──┬──┬──┬──┐    ┌──┬──┬──┬──┬──┐
│▯█│ ★│▲█│ ⊙│★⦅│☟│$ │⁄$│⌸│⊟│ ⊞│⊡│ ⌇│⌇│ ⊟│$1│⌀1│◎│    │▤│▦│ ✓│?│◉│
└──┴──┴──┴──┴──┴──┴──┴──┴──┴──┴──┴──┴──┴──┴──┴──┴──┴──┘    └──┴──┴──┴──┴──┘

Patient #: 319.0    [Wayne Miles                     ]      Dept.  :  0
Voucher #: 1163              Doctor #  :  2 Simpson M.D., Fran  Location :
                            Supervisor:  2 Simpson M.D., Fran
Dates    P.O.S.  Procedure   Modifier Diag. 1-4    Units      Charges   T.O.S.

04/16/03  3       █..........                      .....    $    58.00  1

|X-Ray Chest Pa & Lat             |480.0      Viral Pneumonia
Comment:                          |
                                  |      ..........
                                  |      ..........
Ins: Primary#: 0.0        Assign: .    Secondary#: .......    EMC Billable: .
[Posted]
      Date     Co #  Dr# Procedure   Diag       Units      Charges   Total Chgs

   1  04/16/03      2   99214       480.0        1.00        50.00      50.00
   2  04/16/03      2   85031       480.0        1.00        15.00      65.00
   3  04/16/03      2   71020       480.0        1.00        58.00     123.00



   Enter '?', '!', '?code' for Help, '?~' for Macros, or '%' for Standing Orders

┌
Ready                                          [        ] [       ] [↑↓◁▷]
```

Figure 6-3 Check from Patient – Miles

Wayne and Sheila Miles   1624
40 Kentucky Lane
Madison, CA 95653-0235   *April 16*   20 *03*

Pay to the
order of   *Sydney Carrington & Associates* $ | 123.00 |

         One hundred twenty three and 00/100   Dollars

FIRST COMMUNITY BANK
Madison, California

Memo _____   *Wayne Miles*

⑆04204339⑆ 34274⑈ 1624

Figure 6-4 Payment from Patient

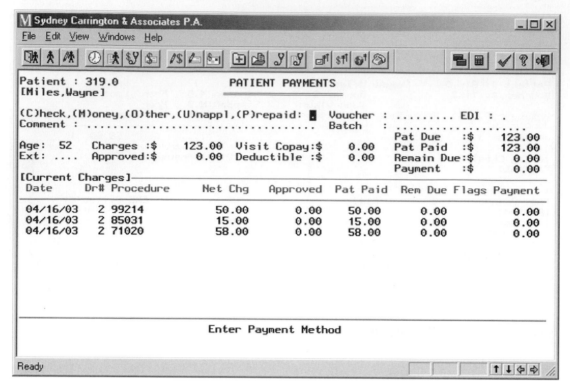

```
M Sydney Carrington & Associates P.A.                                    _ □ X
 File  Edit  View  Windows  Help

  ▦ ⚎ ⚎   ⊙ ⚎ ⚎ $   /$ ⚎ ⚎   ⊞ ⚎ ⚎ ⚎   ⚎ $⚎ ⚎ ⚎        ⚎ ⚎   ✓ ? ⚎

 Patient : 319.0                  PATIENT PAYMENTS
 [Miles,Wayne]

 (C)heck,(M)oney,(O)ther,(U)nappl,(P)repaid: ▮  Voucher : ......... EDI : .
 Comment : ................................   Batch   : .................
                                                     Pat Due   :$    123.00
 Age:  52   Charges :$    123.00  Visit Copay:$   0.00  Pat Paid  :$    123.00
 Ext:  ...  Approved:$      0.00  Deductible :$   0.00  Remain Due:$      0.00
                                                     Payment   :$      0.00
 [Current Charges]──────────────────────────────────────────────────────
  Date      Dr# Procedure      Net Chg   Approved  Pat Paid  Rem Due Flags Payment

  04/16/03   2 99214            50.00      0.00     50.00     0.00          0.00
  04/16/03   2 85031            15.00      0.00     15.00     0.00          0.00
  04/16/03   2 71020            58.00      0.00     58.00     0.00          0.00




 ────────────────────────────────────────────────────────────────────────
                           Enter Payment Method


 Ready                                              ┌──┬──┬──┐ ↑ ↓ ⇦ ⇨
```

EXERCISE 2: PATIENT COPAYMENT

LEANNA RAMIREZ; ACCOUNT 320

GOAL(S): In this exercise you will post procedures and a payment from the Procedure Entry screen for Leanna Ramirez, who will pay a $10 copayment.

1. Before posting your entry, study the encounter form in Figure 6-5 (page 102). Note the charges and diagnosis before attempting the data entry.

2. Based on the information found on the encounter form, post the charges for Leanna Ramirez. Compare your screen to Figure 6-6.

3. Leanna Ramirez provides a check for her $10 copayment. See Figure 6-7. Apply the check for $10 to her account. Compare your screen to Figure 6-8.

Figure 6-5 Encounter Form – Ramirez

Sydney Carrington & Associates P.A.
34 Sycamore Street   Suite 300
Madison, CA 95653

Date: 04/16/2003

Time:

Patient: Leanna Ramirez
Guarantor:

Voucher No.: 1344

Patient No: 320.0

Doctor: 1 - J. Monroe

	CPT	DESCRIPTION	FEE		CPT	DESCRIPTION	FEE		CPT	DESCRIPTION	FEE
OFFICE/HOSPITAL CONSULTS				**LABORATORY/RADIOLOGY**				**PROCEDURES/TESTS**			
☐	99201	Office New:Focused Hx-Exam	___	☐	81000	Urinalysis	___	☐	00452	Anesthesia for Rad Surgery	___
☐	99202	Office New:Expanded Hx-Exam	___	☐	81002	Urinalysis; Pregnancy Test	___	☐	11100	Skin Biopsy	___
☐	99211	Office Estb:Min/None Hx-Exa	___	☐	82951	Glucose Tolerance Test	___	☐	15852	Dressing Change	___
☐	99212	Office Estb:Focused Hx-Exam	___	☐	84478	Triglycerides	___	☐	29075	Cast Appl. - Lower Arm	___
☒	99213	Office Estb:Expanded Hx-Exa	$40	☐	84550	Uric Acid: Blood Chemistry	___	☐	29530	Strapping of Knee	___
☐	99214	Office Estb:Detailed Hx-Exa	___	☐	84830	Ovulation Test	___	☐	29705	Removal/Revis of Cast w/Exa	___
☐	99215	Office Estb:Comprhn Hx-Exam	___	☐	85014	Hematocrit	___	☐	53670	Catheterization Incl. Suppl	___
☐	99221	Hosp. Initial:Comprh Hx-	___	☒	85031	Hemogram, Complete Blood Wk	$15	☐	57452	Colposcopy	___
☐	99223	Hosp.Ini:Comprh Hx-Exam/Hi	___	☐	86403	Particle Agglutination Test	___	☐	57505	ECC	___
☐	99231	Hosp. Subsequent: S-Fwd	___	☐	86485	Skin Test; Candida	___	☐	69420	Myringotomy	___
☐	99232	Hosp. Subsequent: Comprhn Hx	___	☐	86580	TB Intradermal Test	___	☐	92081	Visual Field Examination	___
☐	99233	Hosp. Subsequent: Ex/Hi	___	☐	86585	TB Tine Test	___	☐	92100	Serial Tonometry Exam	___
☐	99238	Hospital Visit Discharge Ex	___	☐	87070	Culture	___	☐	92120	Tonography	___
☐	99371	Telephone Consult - Simple	___	☐	70190	X-Ray; Optic Foramina	___	☐	92552	Pure Tone Audiometry	___
☐	99372	Telephone Consult - Intermed	___	☐	70210	X-Ray Sinuses Complete	___	☐	92567	Tympanometry	___
☐	99373	Telephone Consult - Complex	___	☐	71010	Radiological Exam Ent Spine	___	☐	93000	Electrocardiogram	___
☐	90843	Counseling - 25 minutes	___	☐	71020	X-Ray Chest Pa & Lat	___	☐	93015	Exercise Stress Test (ETT)	___
☐	90844	Counseling - 50 minutes	___	☐	72050	X-Ray Spine, Cerv (4 views)	___	☐	93017	ETT Tracing Only	___
☐	90865	Counseling - Special Interview	___	☐	72090	X-Ray Spine; Scoliosis Ex	___	☐	93040	Electrocardiogram - Rhythm	___
				☐	72110	Spine, lumbosacral; a/p & Lat	___	☐	96100	Psychological Testing	___
IMMUNIZATIONS/INJECTIONS				☐	73030	Shoulder-Comp, min w/ 2vws	___	☐	99000	Specimen Handling	___
☐	90585	BCG Vaccine	___	☐	73070	Elbow, anteropost & later vws	___	☐	99058	Office Emergency Care	___
☐	90659	Influenza Virus Vaccine	___	☐	73120	X-Ray; Hand, 2 views	___	☐	99070	Surgical Tray - Misc.	___
☐	90701	Immunization-DTP	___	☐	73560	X-Ray, Knee, 1 or 2 views	___	☐	99080	Special Reports of Med Rec	___
☐	90702	DT Vaccine	___	☐	74022	X-Ray; Abdomen, Complete	___	☐	99195	Phlebotomy	___
☐	90703	Tetanus Toxoids	___	☐	75552	Cardiac Magnetic Res Img	___	☐	___	_____	___
☐	90732	Pneumococcal Vaccine	___	☐	76020	X-Ray; Bone Age Studies	___	☐	___	_____	___
☐	90746	Hepatitis B Vaccine	___	☐	76088	Mammary Ductogram Complete	___	☐	___	_____	___
☐	90749	Immunization; Unlisted	___	☐	78465	Myocardial Perfusion Img	___	☐	___	_____	___

	ICD-9 CODE DIAGNOSIS			ICD-9 CODE DIAGNOSIS			ICD-9 CODE DIAGNOSIS	
☐	009.0	Ill-defined Intestinal Infect	☐	435.0	Basilar Artery Syndrome	☐	724.2	Pain: Lower Back
☐	133.2	Establish Baseline	☐	440.0	Atherosclerosis	☐	727.6	Rupture of Achilles Tendon
☐	174.9	Breast Cancer	☐	442.81	Carotid Artery	☐	780.1	Hallucinations
☐	185.0	Prostate Cancer	☐	460.0	Common Cold	☐	780.3	Convulsions
☐	250	Diabetes Mellitus	☐	461.9	Acute Sinusitis	☐	780.5	Sleep Disturbances
☐	272.4	Hyperlipidemia	☐	474.0	Tonsillitis	☐	783.0	Anorexia
☐	282.5	Anemia - Sickle Trait	☐	477.9	Hay Fever	☐	783.1	Abnormal Weight Gain
☐	282.60	Anemia - Sickle Cell	☐	487.0	Flu	☐	783.2	Abnormal Weight Loss
☐	285.9	Anemia, Unspecified	☐	496	Chronic Airway Obstruction	☐	830.6	Dislocated Hip
☐	300.4	Neurotic Depression	☐	522	Low Red Blood Count	☐	830.9	Dislocated Shoulder
☐	340	Multiple Sclerosis	☐	524.6	Temporo-Mandibular Jnt Synd	☐	841.2	Sprained Wrist
☐	342.9	Hemiplegia - Unspecified	☐	538.8	Stomach Pain	☐	842.5	Sprained Ankle
☐	346.9	Migraine Headache	☐	553.3	Hiatal Hernia	☐	891.2	Fractured Tibia
☐	352.9	Cranial Neuralgia	☐	564.1	Spastic Colon	☐	892.0	Fractured Fibula
☐	354.0	Carpal Tunnel Syndrome	☐	571.4	Chronic Hepatitis	☐	919.5	Insect Bite, Nonvenomous
☐	355.0	Sciatic Nerve Root Lesion	☐	571.5	Cirrhosis of Liver	☐	921.1	Contus Eyelid/Perioc Area
☐	366.9	Cataract	☐	573.3	Hepatitis	☐	v16.3	Fam. Hist of Breast Cancer
☒	386.0	Vertigo	☐	575.2	Obstruction of Gallbladder	☐	v17.4	Fam. Hist of Cardiovasc Dis
☐	401.1	Essential Hypertension	☐	648.2	Anemia - Compl. Pregnancy	☐	v20.2	Well Child
☐	414.9	Ischemic Hearth Disease	☐	715.90	Osteoarthritis - Unspec	☐	v22.0	Pregnancy - First Normal
☐	428.0	Congestive Heart Failure	☐	721.3	Lumbar Osteo/Spondylarthrit	☐	v22.1	Pregnancy - Normal

Previous Balance	Today's Charges	Total Due	Amount Paid	New Balance
___	___	___	$10 check #1029	___

Follow Up

PRN _____ Weeks _____ Months _____ Units _____

Next Appointment Date: _____   Time: _____

I hereby authorize release of any information acquired in the course of
examination or treatment and allow a photocopy of my signature to be used.

Figure 6-6 Two Procedures Posted – Ramirez

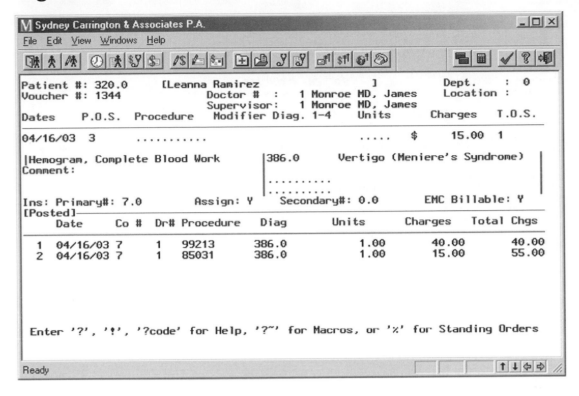

Figure 6-7 Check from Patient – Ramirez

Michael and Leanna Ramirez   1029
25-12 Blossom Street
Sacramento, CA 94056   *April 16*   20 *03*

Pay to the
order of   *Sydney Carrington & Associates* $ | 10.00 |

              Ten and 00/100   Dollars

FIRST COMMUNITY BANK
Madison, California

Memo _____   *Leanna Ramirez*

⑆153154403⑆ 45385⑈ 1029

Figure 6-8 Patient Visit Copay

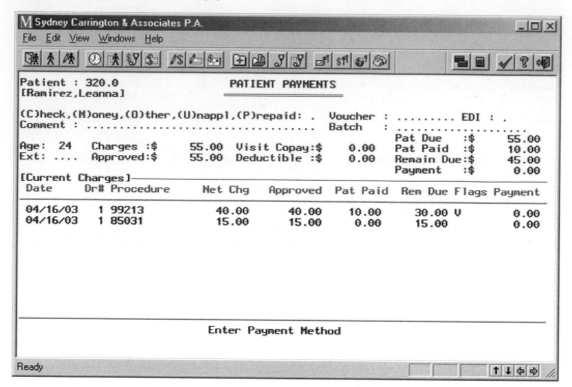

EXERCISE 3: PAYMENT ENTRY

ANNA MARCHESE; ACCOUNT 321

GOAL(S): In this exercise you will post a procedure and post a payment from the Payment Entry screen for Anna Marchese, who will pay in full for her visit.

1. Before posting your entry, study the encounter form in Figure 6-9 (page 106). Note the charge and diagnosis before attempting the data entry.

2. Based on the information found on the encounter form, post the charge for Anna Marchese. Compare your screen to Figure 6-10, then <Process> the screen and exit the Procedure Entry screen.

3. Anna Marchese comes back later that day to give you a check for her visit. See Figure 6-11. Apply the $40 check to her account. Compare your screen to Figure 6-12 before you press the F1 key.

Figure 6-9 Encounter Form – Marchese

Sydney Carrington & Associates P.A.
34 Sycamore Street   Suite 300
Madison, CA 95653

Date: 04/16/2003

Time:

Patient: Anna Marchese
Guarantor:

Voucher No.: 1011

Patient No: 321.0
Doctor: 3 - S. Carrington

	CPT	DESCRIPTION	FEE
		OFFICE/HOSPITAL CONSULTS	
☐	99201	Office New:Focused Hx-Exam	
☐	99202	Office New:Expanded Hx-Exam	
☐	99211	Office Estb:Min/None Hx-Exa	
☐	99212	Office Estb:Focused Hx-Exam	
☒	99213	Office Estb:Expanded Hx-Exa	$40
☐	99214	Office Estb:Detailed Hx-Exa	
☐	99215	Office Estb:Comprhn Hx-Exam	
☐	99221	Hosp. Initial:Comprh Hx-	
☐	99223	Hosp.Ini:Comprh Hx-Exam/Hi	
☐	99231	Hosp. Subsequent: S-Fwd	
☐	99232	Hosp. Subsequent: Comprhn Hx	
☐	99233	Hosp. Subsequent: Ex/Hi	
☐	99238	Hospital Visit Discharge Ex	
☐	99371	Telephone Consult - Simple	
☐	99372	Telephone Consult - Intermed	
☐	99373	Telephone Consult - Complex	
☐	90843	Counseling - 25 minutes	
☐	90844	Counseling - 50 minutes	
☐	90865	Counseling - Special Interview	
		IMMUNIZATIONS/INJECTIONS	
☐	90585	BCG Vaccine	
☐	90659	Influenza Virus Vaccine	
☐	90701	Immunization-DTP	
☐	90702	DT Vaccine	
☐	90703	Tetanus Toxoids	
☐	90732	Pneumococcal Vaccine	
☐	90746	Hepatitis B Vaccine	
☐	90749	Immunization; Unlisted	

	CPT	DESCRIPTION	FEE
		LABORATORY/RADIOLOGY	
☐	81000	Urinalysis	
☐	81002	Urinalysis; Pregnancy Test	
☐	82951	Glucose Tolerance Test	
☐	84478	Triglycerides	
☐	84550	Uric Acid: Blood Chemistry	
☐	84830	Ovulation Test	
☐	85014	Hematocrit	
☐	85031	Hemogram, Complete Blood Wk	
☐	86403	Particle Agglutination Test	
☐	86485	Skin Test; Candida	
☐	86580	TB Intradermal Test	
☐	86585	TB Tine Test	
☐	87070	Culture	
☐	70190	X-Ray; Optic Foramina	
☐	70210	X-Ray Sinuses Complete	
☐	71010	Radiological Exam Ent Spine	
☐	71020	X-Ray Chest Pa & Lat	
☐	72050	X-Ray Spine, Cerv (4 views)	
☐	72090	X-Ray Spine; Scoliosis Ex	
☐	72110	Spine, lumbosacral; a/p & Lat	
☐	73030	Shoulder-Comp, min w/ 2vws	
☐	73070	Elbow, anteropost & later vws	
☐	73120	X-Ray; Hand, 2 views	
☐	73560	X-Ray, Knee, 1 or 2 views	
☐	74022	X-Ray; Abdomen, Complete	
☐	75552	Cardiac Magnetic Res Img	
☐	76020	X-Ray; Bone Age Studies	
☐	76088	Mammary Ductogram Complete	
☐	78465	Myocardial Perfusion Img	

	CPT	DESCRIPTION	FEE
		PROCEDURES/TESTS	
☐	00452	Anesthesia for Rad Surgery	
☐	11100	Skin Biopsy	
☐	15852	Dressing Change	
☐	29075	Cast Appl. - Lower Arm	
☐	29530	Strapping of Knee	
☐	29705	Removal/Revis of Cast w/Exa	
☐	53670	Catheterization Incl. Suppl	
☐	57452	Colposcopy	
☐	57505	ECC	
☐	69420	Myringotomy	
☐	92081	Visual Field Examination	
☐	92100	Serial Tonometry Exam	
☐	92120	Tonography	
☐	92552	Pure Tone Audiometry	
☐	92567	Tympanometry	
☐	93000	Electrocardiogram	
☐	93015	Exercise Stress Test (ETT)	
☐	93017	ETT Tracing Only	
☐	93040	Electrocardiogram - Rhythm	
☐	96100	Psychological Testing	
☐	99000	Specimen Handling	
☐	99058	Office Emergency Care	
☐	99070	Surgical Tray - Misc.	
☐	99080	Special Reports of Med Rec	
☐	99195	Phlebotomy	
☐		_____	
☐		_____	
☐		_____	

		ICD-9 CODE DIAGNOSIS
☐	009.0	Ill-defined Intestinal Infect
☐	133.2	Establish Baseline
☐	174.9	Breast Cancer
☐	185.0	Prostate Cancer
☒	250	Diabetes Mellitus
☐	272.4	Hyperlipidemia
☐	282.5	Anemia - Sickle Trait
☐	282.60	Anemia - Sickle Cell
☐	285.9	Anemia, Unspecified
☐	300.4	Neurotic Depression
☐	340	Multiple Sclerosis
☐	342.9	Hemiplegia - Unspecified
☐	346.9	Migraine Headache
☐	352.9	Cranial Neuralgia
☐	354.0	Carpal Tunnel Syndrome
☐	355.0	Sciatic Nerve Root Lesion
☐	366.9	Cataract
☐	386.0	Vertigo
☐	401.1	Essential Hypertension
☐	414.9	Ischemic Hearth Disease
☐	428.0	Congestive Heart Failure

		ICD-9 CODE DIAGNOSIS
☐	435.0	Basilar Artery Syndrome
☐	440.0	Atherosclerosis
☐	442.81	Carotid Artery
☐	460.0	Common Cold
☒	461.9	Acute Sinusitis
☐	474.0	Tonsillitis
☐	477.9	Hay Fever
☐	487.0	Flu
☐	496	Chronic Airway Obstruction
☐	522	Low Red Blood Count
☐	524.6	Temporo-Mandibular Jnt Synd
☐	538.8	Stomach Pain
☐	553.3	Hiatal Hernia
☐	564.1	Spastic Colon
☐	571.4	Chronic Hepatitis
☐	571.5	Cirrhosis of Liver
☐	573.3	Hepatitis
☐	575.2	Obstruction of Gallbladder
☐	648.2	Anemia - Compl. Pregnancy
☐	715.90	Osteoarthritis - Unspec
☐	721.3	Lumbar Osteo/Spondylarthrit

		ICD-9 CODE DIAGNOSIS
☐	724.2	Pain: Lower Back
☐	727.6	Rupture of Achilles Tendon
☐	780.1	Hallucinations
☐	780.3	Convulsions
☐	780.5	Sleep Disturbances
☐	783.0	Anorexia
☐	783.1	Abnormal Weight Gain
☐	783.2	Abnormal Weight Loss
☐	830.6	Dislocated Hip
☐	830.9	Dislocated Shoulder
☐	841.2	Sprained Wrist
☐	842.5	Sprained Ankle
☐	891.2	Fractured Tibia
☐	892.0	Fractured Fibula
☐	919.5	Insect Bite, Nonvenomous
☐	921.1	Contus Eyelid/Perioc Area
☐	v16.3	Fam. Hist of Breast Cancer
☐	v17.4	Fam. Hist of Cardiovasc Dis
☐	v20.2	Well Child
☐	v22.0	Pregnancy - First Normal
☐	v22.1	Pregnancy - Normal

Previous Balance	Today's Charges	Total Due	Amount Paid	New Balance
_____	_____	_____	$40 check #103	

Follow Up

PRN _____ Weeks _____   Months _____ Units _____

Next Appointment Date: _____   Time: _____

I hereby authorize release of any information acquired in the course of examination or treatment and allow a photocopy of my signature to be used.

Figure 6-10 Procedure Entry – No Insurance

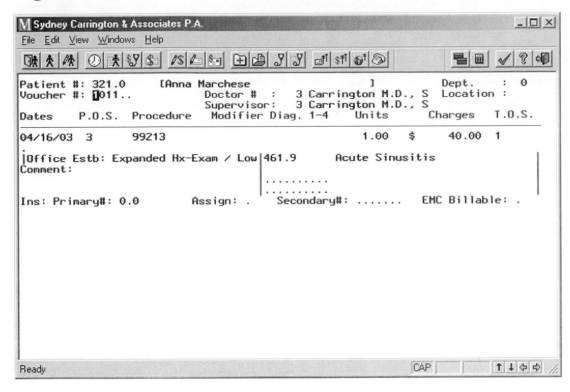

Figure 6-11 Check from Patient – Marchese

Nicholas and Anna Marchese	103
3 Jefferson Avenue	
Floral City, CA 94064	*April 16* 20 *03*

Pay to the
order of _____ *Sydney Carrington & Associates* _____ $ | 40.00 |

Forty and 00/100 _____ Dollars

FIRST COMMUNITY BANK
Madison, California

Memo _____   *Anna Marchese* _____

⑆264265514⑆ 56490⑈ 103

Figure 6-12 Payment Entry Before Posting

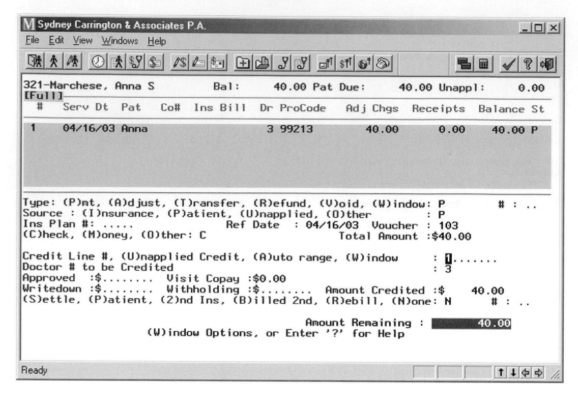

```
M  Sydney Carrington & Associates P.A.                          _ □ ×
 File  Edit  View  Windows  Help

 ⟦▩⟧⟦⟧⟦⟧ ⟦⟧⟦⟧⟦⟧⟦⟧  ⟦⟧⟦⟧⟦⟧  ⟦⟧⟦⟧⟦⟧⟦⟧  ⟦⟧⟦⟧⟦⟧⟦⟧      ⟦⟧⟦⟧ ⟦⟧⟦⟧⟦⟧

321-Marchese, Anna S         Bal:      40.00 Pat Due:    40.00 Unappl:    0.00
[Full]
  #   Serv Dt  Pat   Co#  Ins Bill  Dr ProCode   Adj Chgs  Receipts  Balance St

  1    04/16/03 Anna               3 99213        40.00     0.00     40.00 P




_____
Type: (P)mt, (A)djust, (T)ransfer, (R)efund, (V)oid, (W)indow: P        # : ..
Source : (I)nsurance, (P)atient, (U)napplied, (O)ther       : P
Ins Plan #: .....            Ref Date : 04/16/03  Voucher : 103
(C)heck, (M)oney, (O)ther: C                 Total Amount :$40.00

Credit Line #, (U)napplied Credit, (A)uto range, (W)indow   : 1.......
Doctor # to be Credited                                     : 3
Approved  :$........  Visit Copay :$0.00
Writedown :$........  Withholding :$........  Amount Credited :$   40.00
(S)ettle, (P)atient, (2)nd Ins, (B)illed 2nd, (R)ebill, (N)one: N    # : ..

                              Amount Remaining :      40.00
                 (W)indow Options, or Enter '?' for Help


Ready                                          ⟦⟧⟦⟧  ↑↓⟸⟹
```

EXERCISE 4: APPLYING COPAYMENTS

PAUL SANTOS; CAROL SANTOS; ACCOUNT 322

GOAL(S): In this exercise you will post procedures and post a payment from the Payment Entry screen for Paul and Carol Santos who will pay their copayments.

Paul and Carol Santos have Epsilon insurance and must pay an $8 copayment for each visit. Paul Santos was seen by the doctor early in the day. He left without paying his $8 copayment. Later that same day, Carol Santos was also seen by the doctor. After her visit, she gives a check in the amount of $16 for both of their copayments.

1. Before posting your entry, study the encounter form in Figure 6-13 (page 110). Note the charges and diagnoses before attempting the data entry.

2. Based on the information found on the encounter form, post the charges for Paul Santos. Compare your screen to Figure 6-14, then EXIT the Procedure Entry screen.

Figure 6-13 Encounter Form – Paul Santos

Sydney Carrington & Associates P.A.
34 Sycamore Street   Suite 300
Madison, CA 95653

Date: 04/16/2003

Time:

Patient: Paul Santos
Guarantor:

Voucher No.:   906

Patient No: 322.0
Doctor: 2 - F. Simpson

CPT	DESCRIPTION	FEE
OFFICE/HOSPITAL CONSULTS		
☐ 99201	Office New:Focused Hx-Exam	
☐ 99202	Office New:Expanded Hx-Exam	
☐ 99211	Office Estb:Min/None Hx-Exa	
☐ 99212	Office Estb:Focused Hx-Exam	
☒ 99213	Office Estb:Expanded Hx-Exa	$40
☐ 99214	Office Estb:Detailed Hx-Exa	
☐ 99215	Office Estb:Comprhn Hx-Exam	
☐ 99221	Hosp. Initial:Comprh Hx-	
☐ 99223	Hosp.Ini:Comprh Hx-Exam/Hi	
☐ 99231	Hosp. Subsequent: S-Fwd	
☐ 99232	Hosp. Subsequent: Comprhn Hx	
☐ 99233	Hosp. Subsequent: Ex/Hi	
☐ 99238	Hospital Visit Discharge Ex	
☐ 99371	Telephone Consult - Simple	
☐ 99372	Telephone Consult - Intermed	
☐ 99373	Telephone Consult - Complex	
☐ 90843	Counseling - 25 minutes	
☐ 90844	Counseling - 50 minutes	
☐ 90865	Counseling - Special Interview	
IMMUNIZATIONS/INJECTIONS		
☐ 90585	BCG Vaccine	
☐ 90659	Influenza Virus Vaccine	
☐ 90701	Immunization-DTP	
☐ 90702	DT Vaccine	
☐ 90703	Tetanus Toxoids	
☐ 90732	Pneumococcal Vaccine	
☐ 90746	Hepatitis B Vaccine	
☐ 90749	Immunization; Unlisted	

CPT	DESCRIPTION	FEE
LABORATORY/RADIOLOGY		
☐ 81000	Urinalysis	
☐ 81002	Urinalysis; Pregnancy Test	
☐ 82951	Glucose Tolerance Test	
☐ 84478	Triglycerides	
☐ 84550	Uric Acid: Blood Chemistry	
☐ 84830	Ovulation Test	
☐ 85014	Hematocrit	
☐ 85031	Hemogram, Complete Blood Wk	
☐ 86403	Particle Agglutination Test	
☐ 86485	Skin Test; Candida	
☐ 86580	TB Intradermal Test	
☐ 86585	TB Tine Test	
☐ 87070	Culture	
☐ 70190	X-Ray; Optic Foramina	
☐ 70210	X-Ray Sinuses Complete	
☐ 71010	Radiological Exam Ent Spine	
☐ 71020	X-Ray Chest Pa & Lat	
☐ 72050	X-Ray Spine, Cerv (4 views)	
☐ 72090	X-Ray Spine; Scoliosis Ex	
☐ 72110	Spine, lumbosacral; a/p & Lat	
☐ 73030	Shoulder-Comp, min w/ 2vws	
☐ 73070	Elbow, anteropost & later vws	
☐ 73120	X-Ray; Hand, 2 views	
☐ 73560	X-Ray, Knee, 1 or 2 views	
☐ 74022	X-Ray; Abdomen, Complete	
☐ 75552	Cardiac Magnetic Res Img	
☐ 76020	X-Ray; Bone Age Studies	
☐ 76088	Mammary Ductogram Complete	
☐ 78465	Myocardial Perfusion Img	

CPT	DESCRIPTION	FEE
PROCEDURES/TESTS		
☐ 00452	Anesthesia for Rad Surgery	
☐ 11100	Skin Biopsy	
☐ 15852	Dressing Change	
☐ 29075	Cast Appl. - Lower Arm	
☐ 29530	Strapping of Knee	
☐ 29705	Removal/Revis of Cast w/Exa	
☐ 53670	Catheterization Incl. Suppl	
☐ 57452	Colposcopy	
☐ 57505	ECC	
☐ 69420	Myringotomy	
☐ 92081	Visual Field Examination	
☐ 92100	Serial Tonometry Exam	
☐ 92120	Tonography	
☐ 92552	Pure Tone Audiometry	
☐ 92567	Tympanometry	
☒ 93000	Electrocardiogram	$57
☐ 93015	Exercise Stress Test (ETT)	
☐ 93017	ETT Tracing Only	
☐ 93040	Electrocardiogram - Rhythm	
☐ 96100	Psychological Testing	
☐ 99000	Specimen Handling	
☐ 99058	Office Emergency Care	
☐ 99070	Surgical Tray - Misc.	
☐ 99080	Special Reports of Med Rec	
☐ 99195	Phlebotomy	
☐		
☐		
☐		

ICD-9 CODE DIAGNOSIS	
☐ 009.0	Ill-defined Intestinal Infect
☐ 133.2	Establish Baseline
☐ 174.9	Breast Cancer
☐ 185.0	Prostate Cancer
☐ 250	Diabetes Mellitus
☐ 272.4	Hyperlipidemia
☐ 282.5	Anemia - Sickle Trait
☐ 282.60	Anemia - Sickle Cell
☐ 285.9	Anemia, Unspecified
☐ 300.4	Neurotic Depression
☐ 340	Multiple Sclerosis
☐ 342.9	Hemiplegia - Unspecified
☐ 346.9	Migraine Headache
☐ 352.9	Cranial Neuralgia
☐ 354.0	Carpal Tunnel Syndrome
☐ 355.0	Sciatic Nerve Root Lesion
☐ 366.9	Cataract
☐ 386.0	Vertigo
☐ 401.1	Essential Hypertension
☐ 414.9	Ischemic Hearth Disease
☐ 428.0	Congestive Heart Failure

ICD-9 CODE DIAGNOSIS	
☐ 435.0	Basilar Artery Syndrome
☐ 440.0	Atherosclerosis
☐ 442.81	Carotid Artery
☐ 460.0	Common Cold
☐ 461.9	Acute Sinusitis
☐ 474.0	Tonsillitis
☐ 477.9	Hay Fever
☐ 487.0	Flu
☐ 496	Chronic Airway Obstruction
☐ 522	Low Red Blood Count
☐ 524.6	Temporo-Mandibular Jnt Synd
☐ 538.8	Stomach Pain
☐ 553.3	Hiatal Hernia
☐ 564.1	Spastic Colon
☐ 571.4	Chronic Hepatitis
☐ 571.5	Cirrhosis of Liver
☐ 573.3	Hepatitis
☐ 575.2	Obstruction of Gallbladder
☐ 648.2	Anemia - Compl. Pregnancy
☐ 715.90	Osteoarthritis - Unspec
☐ 721.3	Lumbar Osteo/Spondylarthrit

ICD-9 CODE DIAGNOSIS	
☐ 724.2	Pain: Lower Back
☐ 727.6	Rupture of Achilles Tendon
☐ 780.1	Hallucinations
☐ 780.3	Convulsions
☐ 780.5	Sleep Disturbances
☐ 783.0	Anorexia
☐ 783.1	Abnormal Weight Gain
☐ 783.2	Abnormal Weight Loss
☐ 830.6	Dislocated Hip
☐ 830.9	Dislocated Shoulder
☐ 841.2	Sprained Wrist
☐ 842.5	Sprained Ankle
☐ 891.2	Fractured Tibia
☐ 892.0	Fractured Fibula
☐ 919.5	Insect Bite, Nonvenomous
☐ 921.1	Contus Eyelid/Perioc Area
☐ v16.3	Fam. Hist of Breast Cancer
☐ v17.4	Fam. Hist of Cardiovasc Dis
☐ v20.2	Well Child
☐ v22.0	Pregnancy - First Normal
☐ v22.1	Pregnancy - Normal
X 786.50	Chest Pain

Previous Balance	Today's Charges	Total Due	Amount Paid	New Balance

Follow Up

PRN _____ Weeks _____ Months _____ Units _____

Next Appointment Date: _____   Time: _____

I hereby authorize release of any information acquired in the course of examination or treatment and allow a photocopy of my signature to be used.

Figure 6-14 Posted Procedures – Santos

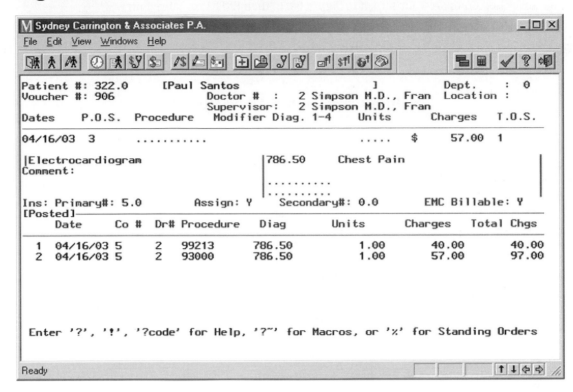

3. Select Carol Santos and based on the information on her encounter form (Figure 6-15), post one charge for her. Compare your screen to Figure 6-16, then EXIT Procedure Entry.

Figure 6-15 Encounter Form – Carol Santos

Sydney Carrington & Associates P.A.
34 Sycamore Street   Suite 300
Madison, CA 95653

Date: 04/16/2003

Time:

Patient: Carol Santos
Guarantor:

Voucher No.: 1215

Patient No: 322.1
Doctor: 2 - F. Simpson

	CPT	DESCRIPTION	FEE		CPT	DESCRIPTION	FEE		CPT	DESCRIPTION	FEE
OFFICE/HOSPITAL CONSULTS				**LABORATORY/RADIOLOGY**				**PROCEDURES/TESTS**			
☐	99201	Office New:Focused Hx-Exam		☐	81000	Urinalysis		☐	00452	Anesthesia for Rad Surgery	
☐	99202	Office New:Expanded Hx-Exam		☐	81002	Urinalysis; Pregnancy Test		☐	11100	Skin Biopsy	
☐	99211	Office Estb:Min/None Hx-Exa		☐	82951	Glucose Tolerance Test		☐	15852	Dressing Change	
☐	99212	Office Estb:Focused Hx-Exam		☐	84478	Triglycerides		☐	29075	Cast Appl. - Lower Arm	
☐	99213	Office Estb:Expanded Hx-Exa		☐	84550	Uric Acid: Blood Chemistry		☐	29530	Strapping of Knee	
☒	99214	Office Estb:Detailed Hx-Exa	$50	☐	84830	Ovulation Test		☐	29705	Removal/Revis of Cast w/Exa	
☐	99215	Office Estb:Comprhn Hx-Exam		☐	85014	Hematocrit		☐	53670	Catheterization Incl. Suppl	
☐	99221	Hosp. Initial:Comprh Hx-		☐	85031	Hemogram, Complete Blood Wk		☐	57452	Colposcopy	
☐	99223	Hosp.Ini:Comprh Hx-Exam/Hi		☐	86403	Particle Agglutination Test		☐	57505	ECC	
☐	99231	Hosp. Subsequent: S-Fwd		☐	86485	Skin Test; Candida		☐	69420	Myringotomy	
☐	99232	Hosp. Subsequent: Comprhn Hx		☐	86580	TB Intradermal Test		☐	92081	Visual Field Examination	
☐	99233	Hosp. Subsequent: Ex/Hi		☐	86585	TB Tine Test		☐	92100	Serial Tonometry Exam	
☐	99238	Hospital Visit Discharge Ex		☐	87070	Culture		☐	92120	Tonography	
☐	99371	Telephone Consult - Simple		☐	70190	X-Ray; Optic Foramina		☐	92552	Pure Tone Audiometry	
☐	99372	Telephone Consult - Intermed		☐	70210	X-Ray Sinuses Complete		☐	92567	Tympanometry	
☐	99373	Telephone Consult - Complex		☐	71010	Radiological Exam Ent Spine		☐	93000	Electrocardiogram	
☐	90843	Counseling - 25 minutes		☐	71020	X-Ray Chest Pa & Lat		☐	93015	Exercise Stress Test (ETT)	
☐	90844	Counseling - 50 minutes		☐	72050	X-Ray Spine, Cerv (4 views)		☐	93017	ETT Tracing Only	
☐	90865	Counseling - Special Interview		☐	72090	X-Ray Spine; Scoliosis Ex		☐	93040	Electrocardiogram - Rhythm	
				☐	72110	Spine, lumbosacral; a/p & Lat		☐	96100	Psychological Testing	
IMMUNIZATIONS/INJECTIONS				☐	73030	Shoulder-Comp, min w/ 2vws		☐	99000	Specimen Handling	
☐	90585	BCG Vaccine		☐	73070	Elbow, anteropost & later vws		☐	99058	Office Emergency Care	
☐	90659	Influenza Virus Vaccine		☐	73120	X-Ray; Hand, 2 views		☐	99070	Surgical Tray - Misc.	
☐	90701	Immunization-DTP		☐	73560	X-Ray, Knee, 1 or 2 views		☐	99080	Special Reports of Med Rec	
☐	90702	DT Vaccine		☐	74022	X-Ray; Abdomen, Complete		☐	99195	Phlebotomy	
☐	90703	Tetanus Toxoids		☐	75552	Cardiac Magnetic Res Img		☐		_____	
☐	90732	Pneumococcal Vaccine		☐	76020	X-Ray; Bone Age Studies		☐		_____	
☐	90746	Hepatitis B Vaccine		☐	76088	Mammary Ductogram Complete		☐		_____	
☐	90749	Immunization; Unlisted		☐	78465	Myocardial Perfusion Img		☐		_____	

	ICD-9 CODE DIAGNOSIS			ICD-9 CODE DIAGNOSIS			ICD-9 CODE DIAGNOSIS	
☐	009.0	Ill-defined Intestinal Infect	☐	435.0	Basilar Artery Syndrome	☐	724.2	Pain: Lower Back
☐	133.2	Establish Baseline	☐	440.0	Atherosclerosis	☐	727.6	Rupture of Achilles Tendon
☐	174.9	Breast Cancer	☐	442.81	Carotid Artery	☐	780.1	Hallucinations
☐	185.0	Prostate Cancer	☐	460.0	Common Cold	☐	780.3	Convulsions
☐	250	Diabetes Mellitus	☐	461.9	Acute Sinusitis	☐	780.5	Sleep Disturbances
☐	272.4	Hyperlipidemia	☐	474.0	Tonsillitis	☐	783.0	Anorexia
☐	282.5	Anemia - Sickle Trait	☐	477.9	Hay Fever	☐	783.1	Abnormal Weight Gain
☐	282.60	Anemia - Sickle Cell	☐	487.0	Flu	☐	783.2	Abnormal Weight Loss
☐	285.9	Anemia, Unspecified	☐	496	Chronic Airway Obstruction	☐	830.6	Dislocated Hip
☐	300.4	Neurotic Depression	☐	522	Low Red Blood Count	☐	830.9	Dislocated Shoulder
☐	340	Multiple Sclerosis	☐	524.6	Temporo-Mandibular Jnt Synd	☐	841.2	Sprained Wrist
☐	342.9	Hemiplegia - Unspecified	☐	538.8	Stomach Pain	☐	842.5	Sprained Ankle
☒	346.9	Migraine Headache	☐	553.3	Hiatal Hernia	☐	891.2	Fractured Tibia
☐	352.9	Cranial Neuralgia	☐	564.1	Spastic Colon	☐	892.0	Fractured Fibula
☐	354.0	Carpal Tunnel Syndrome	☐	571.4	Chronic Hepatitis	☐	919.5	Insect Bite, Nonvenomous
☐	355.0	Sciatic Nerve Root Lesion	☐	571.5	Cirrhosis of Liver	☐	921.1	Contus Eyelid/Perioc Area
☐	366.9	Cataract	☐	573.3	Hepatitis	☐	v16.3	Fam. Hist of Breast Cancer
☐	386.0	Vertigo	☐	575.2	Obstruction of Gallbladder	☐	v17.4	Fam. Hist of Cardiovasc Dis
☐	401.1	Essential Hypertension	☐	648.2	Anemia - Compl. Pregnancy	☐	v20.2	Well Child
☐	414.9	Ischemic Hearth Disease	☐	715.90	Osteoarthritis - Unspec	☐	v22.0	Pregnancy - First Normal
☐	428.0	Congestive Heart Failure	☐	721.3	Lumbar Osteo/Spondylarthrit	☐	v22.1	Pregnancy - Normal

Previous Balance	Today's Charges	Total Due	Amount Paid	New Balance
_____	_____	_____	_____	_____

Follow Up

PRN _____ Weeks _____ Months _____ Units _____

Next Appointment Date: Time:

I hereby authorize release of any information acquired in the course of examination or treatment and allow a photocopy of my signature to be used.

Figure 6-16 Procedure Entry – Carol Santos

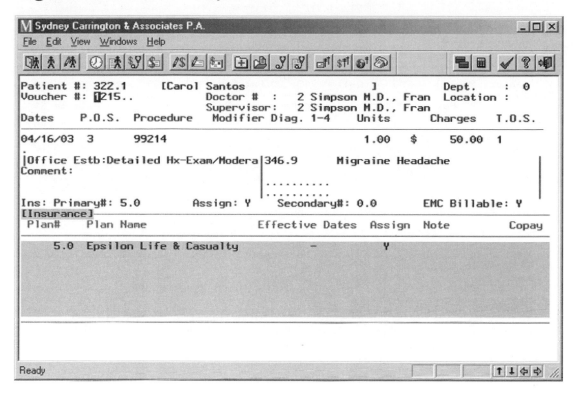

Since Carol Santos is giving a check for $16 (Figure 6-17), which includes her husband's visit copayment, you will need to go to the Payment Entry screen and apply the payment.

4. Apply the $16 check to the account by applying $8 to Paul's office visit and $8 to Carol's office visit. After you have applied the proper amount to all three items, compare your screen to Figure 6-18.

Figure 6-17 Copayment from Paul and Carol Santos

Paul and Carol Santos		1112
105 Crescent Street		
Madison, CA 95653-0235	*April 16*	20 *03*

Pay to the
order of _____*Sydney Carrington & Associates*_____ $ | 16.00 |

_____*Sixteen and 00/100*_____ Dollars

FIRST COMMUNITY BANK
Madison, California

Memo _____ *Carol Santos*

⑅375376625⑅ 67501⑞ 1112

Figure 6-18 Payment Screen After Copay Applied

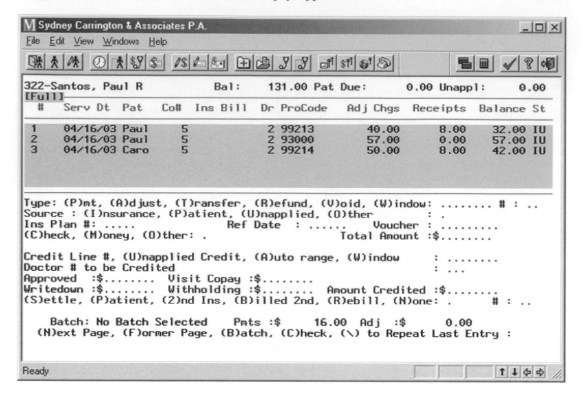

```
M Sydney Carrington & Associates P.A.                              _ □ ×
File  Edit  View  Windows  Help

322-Santos, Paul R            Bal:    131.00 Pat Due:    0.00 Unappl:    0.00
[Full]
 #   Serv Dt  Pat   Co#  Ins Bill  Dr ProCode   Adj Chgs   Receipts   Balance St

 1   04/16/03 Paul    5            2 99213        40.00      8.00      32.00 IU
 2   04/16/03 Paul    5            2 93000        57.00      0.00      57.00 IU
 3   04/16/03 Caro    5            2 99214        50.00      8.00      42.00 IU




Type: (P)mt, (A)djust, (T)ransfer, (R)efund, (V)oid, (W)indow: ........ # : ..
Source : (I)nsurance, (P)atient, (U)napplied, (O)ther        : .
Ins Plan #: .....            Ref Date  : ......      Voucher  : ........
(C)heck, (M)oney, (O)ther: .                   Total Amount :$........

Credit Line #, (U)napplied Credit, (A)uto range, (W)indow    : ........
Doctor # to be Credited                                      : ...
Approved  :$........   Visit Copay :$........
Writedown :$........   Withholding :$........   Amount Credited :$........
(S)ettle, (P)atient, (2)nd Ins, (B)illed 2nd, (R)ebill, (N)one: .       # : ..

    Batch: No Batch Selected     Pmts :$    16.00  Adj :$    0.00
    (N)ext Page, (F)ormer Page, (B)atch, (C)heck, (\) to Repeat Last Entry :

Ready                                                    ↑ ↓ ⇦ ⇨
```

EXERCISE 5: USING AUTO PAY

STEPHEN WEILAND; ACCOUNT 323

GOAL(S): In this exercise you will post charges and post a payment using automatic crediting.

1. Before posting your entry, study the encounter form in Figure 6-19 (page 116). Answer the following questions:

   a. How many procedures were performed? _____

   b. What is the diagnosis? _____

   c. What is the total charge for this visit? _____

Figure 6-19 Encounter Form – Weiland

Sydney Carrington & Associates P.A.
34 Sycamore Street   Suite 300
Madison, CA 95653

Date: 04/16/2003

Voucher No.: 1544

Time:

Patient: Stephen Weiland
Guarantor:

Patient No: 323.1
Doctor: 3 - S. Carrington

	CPT	DESCRIPTION	FEE
		OFFICE/HOSPITAL CONSULTS	
☐	99201	Office New:Focused Hx-Exam	
☐	99202	Office New:Expanded Hx-Exam	
☐	99211	Office Estb:Min/None Hx-Exa	
☐	99212	Office Estb:Focused Hx-Exam	
☐	99213	Office Estb:Expanded Hx-Exa	
☒	99214	Office Estb:Detailed Hx-Exa	$50
☐	99215	Office Estb:Comprhn Hx-Exam	
☐	99221	Hosp. Initial:Comprh Hx-	
☐	99223	Hosp.Ini:Comprh Hx-Exam/Hi	
☐	99231	Hosp. Subsequent: S-Fwd	
☐	99232	Hosp. Subsequent: Comprhn Hx	
☐	99233	Hosp. Subsequent: Ex/Hi	
☐	99238	Hospital Visit Discharge Ex	
☐	99371	Telephone Consult - Simple	
☐	99372	Telephone Consult - Intermed	
☐	99373	Telephone Consult - Complex	
☐	90843	Counseling - 25 minutes	
☐	90844	Counseling - 50 minutes	
☐	90865	Counseling - Special Interview	
		IMMUNIZATIONS/INJECTIONS	
☐	90585	BCG Vaccine	
☐	90659	Influenza Virus Vaccine	
☐	90701	Immunization-DTP	
☐	90702	DT Vaccine	
☐	90703	Tetanus Toxoids	
☐	90732	Pneumococcal Vaccine	
☐	90746	Hepatitis B Vaccine	
☒	90749	Immunization; Unlisted	$12

	CPT	DESCRIPTION	FEE
		LABORATORY/RADIOLOGY	
☒	81000	Urinalysis	$8
☐	81002	Urinalysis; Pregnancy Test	
☐	82951	Glucose Tolerance Test	
☐	84478	Triglycerides	
☐	84550	Uric Acid: Blood Chemistry	
☐	84830	Ovulation Test	
☒	85014	Hematocrit	$18
☐	85031	Hemogram, Complete Blood Wk	
☐	86403	Particle Agglutination Test	
☐	86485	Skin Test; Candida	
☐	86580	TB Intradermal Test	
☐	86585	TB Tine Test	
☐	87070	Culture	
☐	70190	X-Ray; Optic Foramina	
☐	70210	X-Ray Sinuses Complete	
☐	71010	Radiological Exam Ent Spine	
☐	71020	X-Ray Chest Pa & Lat	
☐	72050	X-Ray Spine, Cerv (4 views)	
☐	72090	X-Ray Spine; Scoliosis Ex	
☐	72110	Spine, lumbosacral; a/p & Lat	
☐	73030	Shoulder-Comp, min w/ 2vws	
☐	73070	Elbow, anteropost & later vws	
☐	73120	X-Ray; Hand, 2 views	
☐	73560	X-Ray, Knee, 1 or 2 views	
☐	74022	X-Ray; Abdomen, Complete	
☐	75552	Cardiac Magnetic Res Img	
☐	76020	X-Ray; Bone Age Studies	
☐	76088	Mammary Ductogram Complete	
☐	78465	Myocardial Perfusion Img	

	CPT	DESCRIPTION	FEE
		PROCEDURES/TESTS	
☐	00452	Anesthesia for Rad Surgery	
☐	11100	Skin Biopsy	
☐	15852	Dressing Change	
☐	29075	Cast Appl. - Lower Arm	
☐	29530	Strapping of Knee	
☐	29705	Removal/Revis of Cast w/Exa	
☐	53670	Catheterization Incl. Suppl	
☐	57452	Colposcopy	
☐	57505	ECC	
☐	69420	Myringotomy	
☐	92081	Visual Field Examination	
☐	92100	Serial Tonometry Exam	
☐	92120	Tonography	
☐	92552	Pure Tone Audiometry	
☐	92567	Tympanometry	
☐	93000	Electrocardiogram	
☐	93015	Exercise Stress Test (ETT)	
☐	93017	ETT Tracing Only	
☐	93040	Electrocardiogram - Rhythm	
☐	96100	Psychological Testing	
☐	99000	Specimen Handling	
☐	99058	Office Emergency Care	
☐	99070	Surgical Tray - Misc.	
☐	99080	Special Reports of Med Rec	
☐	99195	Phlebotomy	
☐			
☐			
☐			

	ICD-9 CODE DIAGNOSIS	
☐	009.0	Ill-defined Intestinal Infect
☐	133.2	Establish Baseline
☐	174.9	Breast Cancer
☐	185.0	Prostate Cancer
☐	250	Diabetes Mellitus
☐	272.4	Hyperlipidemia
☐	282.5	Anemia - Sickle Trait
☐	282.60	Anemia - Sickle Cell
☐	285.9	Anemia, Unspecified
☐	300.4	Neurotic Depression
☐	340	Multiple Sclerosis
☐	342.9	Hemiplegia - Unspecified
☐	346.9	Migraine Headache
☐	352.9	Cranial Neuralgia
☐	354.0	Carpal Tunnel Syndrome
☐	355.0	Sciatic Nerve Root Lesion
☐	366.9	Cataract
☐	386.0	Vertigo
☐	401.1	Essential Hypertension
☐	414.9	Ischemic Hearth Disease
☐	428.0	Congestive Heart Failure

	ICD-9 CODE DIAGNOSIS	
☐	435.0	Basilar Artery Syndrome
☐	440.0	Atherosclerosis
☐	442.81	Carotid Artery
☐	460.0	Common Cold
☐	461.9	Acute Sinusitis
☐	474.0	Tonsillitis
☐	477.9	Hay Fever
☐	487.0	Flu
☐	496	Chronic Airway Obstruction
☐	522	Low Red Blood Count
☐	524.6	Temporo-Mandibular Jnt Synd
☐	538.8	Stomach Pain
☐	553.3	Hiatal Hernia
☐	564.1	Spastic Colon
☐	571.4	Chronic Hepatitis
☐	571.5	Cirrhosis of Liver
☐	573.3	Hepatitis
☐	575.2	Obstruction of Gallbladder
☐	648.2	Anemia - Compl. Pregnancy
☐	715.90	Osteoarthritis - Unspec
☐	721.3	Lumbar Osteo/Spondylarthrit

	ICD-9 CODE DIAGNOSIS	
☐	724.2	Pain: Lower Back
☐	727.6	Rupture of Achilles Tendon
☐	780.1	Hallucinations
☐	780.3	Convulsions
☐	780.5	Sleep Disturbances
☐	783.0	Anorexia
☐	783.1	Abnormal Weight Gain
☐	783.2	Abnormal Weight Loss
☐	830.6	Dislocated Hip
☐	830.9	Dislocated Shoulder
☐	841.2	Sprained Wrist
☐	842.5	Sprained Ankle
☐	891.2	Fractured Tibia
☐	892.0	Fractured Fibula
☐	919.5	Insect Bite, Nonvenomous
☐	921.1	Contus Eyelid/Perioc Area
☐	v16.3	Fam. Hist of Breast Cancer
☐	v17.4	Fam. Hist of Cardiovasc Dis
☒	v20.2	Well Child
☐	v22.0	Pregnancy - First Normal
☐	v22.1	Pregnancy - Normal

Previous Balance	Today's Charges	Total Due	Amount Paid	New Balance
			$88 check #427	

Follow Up

PRN _____ Weeks _____   Months _____ Units _____

Next Appointment Date: Time:

I hereby authorize release of any information acquired in the course of examination or treatment and allow a photocopy of my signature to be used.

2. Based on the information found on the encounter form, post the charges for Stephen Weiland. After you have posted three of the four charges, compare your screen to Figure 6-20.

3. Post the payment (Figure 6-21) from the Payment Entry screen, using the automatic crediting feature. Compare your screen to Figure 6-22 before you press the F1 key. Compare your screen to Figure 6-23 after you have pressed the F1 key.

Figure 6-20 Four Procedures Posted – Weiland

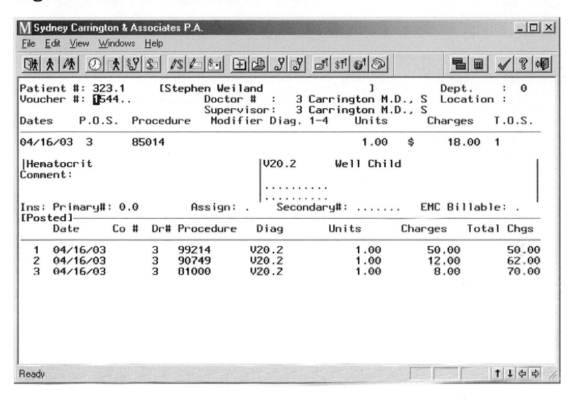

Figure 6-21 Check from Patient – Weiland

Candace Weiland   427
13-48 Kleinfeld Avenue
Madison, CA 95653-0609   *April 16*   20 *03*

Pay to the
order of _____ *Sydney Carrington & Associates* _____ $ | 88.00 |

                    Eighty eight and 00/100   Dollars

FIRST COMMUNITY BANK
Madison, California

Memo _____   *Candace Weiland*

⑈486487736⑈ 786 12⑈ 427

Figure 6-22 Payment Screen Before Posting

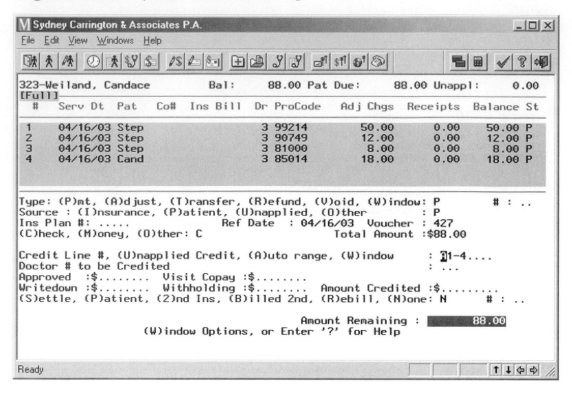

Figure 6-23 Payment Screen After Posting

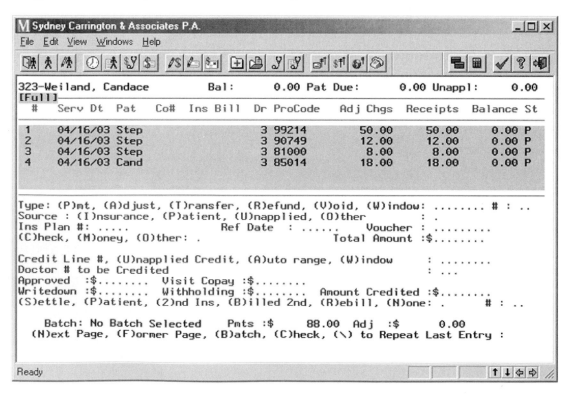

EXERCISE 6: POSTING INSURANCE PAYMENT SPLIT BETWEEN PATIENTS

GOAL(S): Apply the insurance check from Pan American to four different patient accounts. You will bill secondary insurances and use the settlement option.

Insurance plan #7, Pan American, sends check 584121 for $444.82. (See Figure 6-24.) The check is to be split between four patient accounts. The Explanation of Benefits indicates the payment allocations for each charge. In some cases you will settle the remaining balances, and others you will bill the secondary insurance plan.

Figure 6-24 Explanation of Benefits

PAN AMERICAN	584121
259 Anchorage Avenue	Bank of America
San Diego, CA 96588	Palo Alto, CA 96344
	Date: 04/16/03

PAY FOUR HUNDRED FORTY FOUR AND 83/100.......DOLLARS $444.82

TO   SYDNEY CARRINGTON, MD

THE   34 Sycamore Street

ORDER   Madison,CA 95653

OF

100911199 08 324411778: 03

04/16/03

Pan American Insurance Company
Explanation of Benefits

Provider: Sydney Carrington, MD   Provider #: 1155123
              34 Sycamore Street
              Madison, CA 95653

ID/Patient	Service Date	CPT	POS	TOS	Units	Chg	Copay	Paid	
463127934	020103	99214	03	01	1	50.00	10.00	32.48	
Hatcher, Craig	020103	81000	03	01	1	8.00	0.00	6.23	
	020103	85031	03	01	1	15.00	0.00	12.64	
							Total	51.35	
PX671352	020103	99215	03	01	1	85.00	8.00	70.45	
Roberts, Ashleigh	020103	81000	03	01	1	8.00	0.00	6.23	
							Total	76.68	
781356	020103	99215	03	01	1	85.00	15.00	59.72	
Scheller, Denise	020103	81000	03	01	1	8.00	0.00	6.23	
	020103	85014	03	01	1	18.00	0.00	16.84	
	020103	85031	03	01	1	15.00	0.00	12.64	
							Total	95.43	
461461461	020103	99215	03	01	1	85.00	2.00	76.34	
Fitzpatrick, Mark	020103	81000	03	01	1	8.00	0.00	6.23	
	020103	72050	03	01	1	150.00	0.00	138.79	
							Total	221.36	

NOTE: After choosing to settle or bill the secondary insurance plan, you will be warned that the item is pending insurance billing. For the purposes of this exercise, choose 'Y' to continue.

1. Before posting your entry, study the explanation of benefits in Figure 6-24. Answer the following questions:

   a. What patient accounts are being paid by Pan American? _____

   b. What are the total payments for each account? _____

   c. What are the service dates that are being paid by Pan American? _____

3. Based on the information found on the explanation of benefits, post the payments for each patient separately. Enter the total paid for each patient as the amount of the check for that patient. Apply the amounts for each line exactly as shown. For each patient, compare your screen to the figure before posting the first payment and the figure after the successful posting of all items for that patient.

Figure 6-25   Before Posting First Item – Hatcher

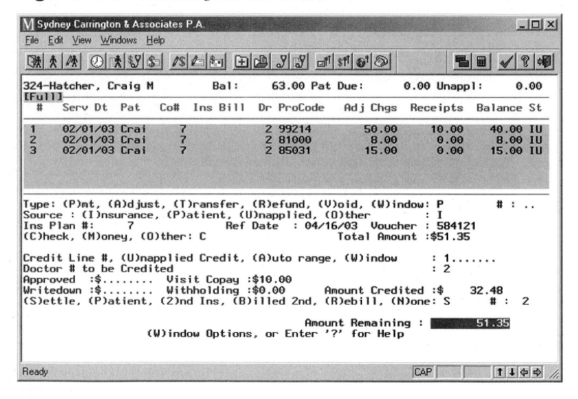

Figure 6-26 After Posting Last Item – Hatcher

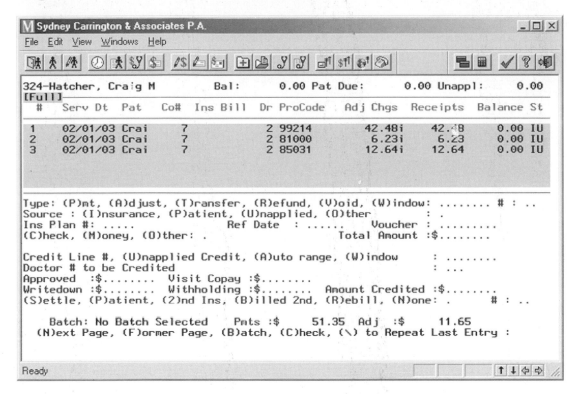

```
M  Sydney Carrington & Associates P.A.                              _ □ ×
   File  Edit  View  Windows  Help

   [toolbar icons]                                      [toolbar icons]

   324-Hatcher, Craig M        Bal:      0.00 Pat Due:      0.00 Unappl:    0.00
   [Full]
    #   Serv Dt   Pat   Co#  Ins Bill  Dr ProCode  Adj Chgs  Receipts  Balance St

    1   02/01/03  Crai   7              2 99214       42.48i    42.48     0.00 IU
    2   02/01/03  Crai   7              2 81000        6.23i     6.23     0.00 IU
    3   02/01/03  Crai   7              2 85031       12.64i    12.64     0.00 IU


   Type: (P)mt, (A)djust, (T)ransfer, (R)efund, (V)oid, (W)indow: ........ # : ..
   Source : (I)nsurance, (P)atient, (U)napplied, (O)ther      : .
   Ins Plan #: .....              Ref Date  : ......   Voucher : ...........
   (C)heck, (M)oney, (O)ther: .                  Total Amount :$........

   Credit Line #, (U)napplied Credit, (A)uto range, (W)indow   : ........
   Doctor # to be Credited                                     : ...
   Approved  :$........  Visit Copay :$........
   Writedown :$........  Withholding :$........   Amount Credited :$........
   (S)ettle, (P)atient, (2)nd Ins, (B)illed 2nd, (R)ebill, (N)one: .     # : ..

       Batch: No Batch Selected    Pmts :$     51.35  Adj :$     11.65
       (N)ext Page, (F)ormer Page, (B)atch, (C)heck, (\) to Repeat Last Entry :

   Ready                                                   ↑ ↓ ⇔ ⇨
```

Figure 6-27 Before Posting First Item – Roberts

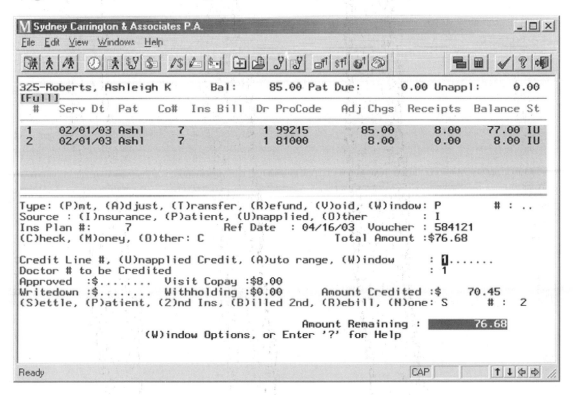

```
M  Sydney Carrington & Associates P.A.                              _ □ ×
   File  Edit  View  Windows  Help

   [toolbar icons]                                      [toolbar icons]

   325-Roberts, Ashleigh K     Bal:     85.00 Pat Due:      0.00 Unappl:    0.00
   [Full]
    #   Serv Dt   Pat   Co#  Ins Bill  Dr ProCode  Adj Chgs  Receipts  Balance St

    1   02/01/03  Ashl   7              1 99215       85.00      8.00    77.00 IU
    2   02/01/03  Ashl   7              1 81000        8.00      0.00     8.00 IU


   Type: (P)mt, (A)djust, (T)ransfer, (R)efund, (V)oid, (W)indow: P      # : ..
   Source : (I)nsurance, (P)atient, (U)napplied, (O)ther      : I
   Ins Plan #:    7               Ref Date  : 04/16/03  Voucher : 584121
   (C)heck, (M)oney, (O)ther: C                  Total Amount :$76.68

   Credit Line #, (U)napplied Credit, (A)uto range, (W)indow   : 1.......
   Doctor # to be Credited                                     : 1
   Approved  :$........  Visit Copay :$8.00
   Writedown :$........  Withholding :$0.00     Amount Credited :$    70.45
   (S)ettle, (P)atient, (2)nd Ins, (B)illed 2nd, (R)ebill, (N)one: S    # :  2

                           Amount Remaining :  [  76.68  ]
           (W)indow Options, or Enter '?' for Help

   Ready                                      CAP              ↑ ↓ ⇔ ⇨
```

Figure 6-28 After Posting Last Item – Roberts

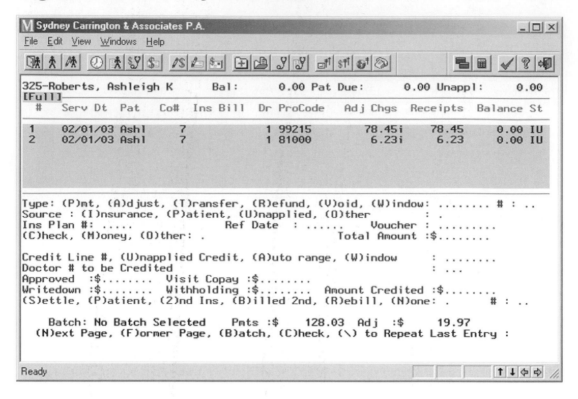

Figure 6-29 Before Posting First Item – Scheller

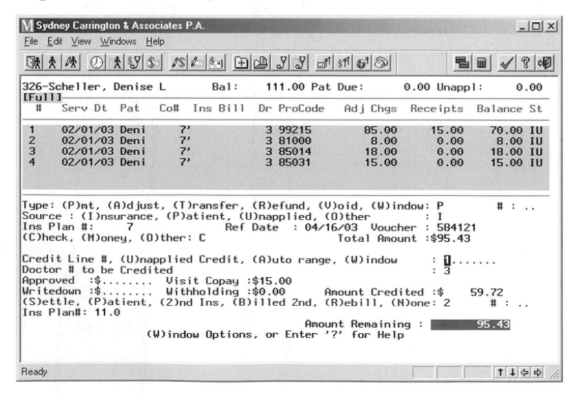

Figure 6-30 After Posting Last Item – Scheller

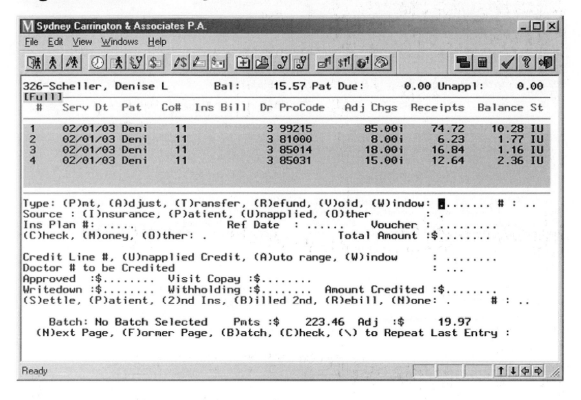

Figure 6-31 Before Posting First Item – Fitzpatrick

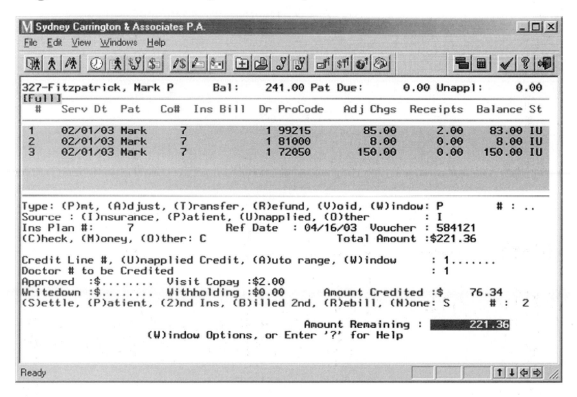

Figure 6-32 After Posting Last Item – Fitzpatrick

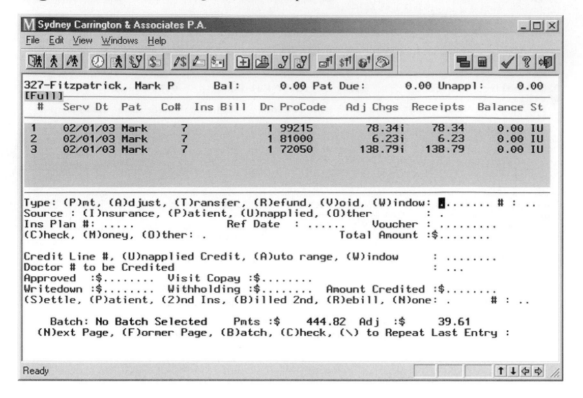

U N I T 7

Report Generation

In the unit exercises that follow, you will generate a Guarantors' Financial Summary report, Current Period report, and System Financial Summary report and print patient statements.

*NOTE: **The reports will be based on the account activity entered to date. Therefore, the report information will vary by the unit exercises that have been completed.***

EXERCISE 1: GUARANTORS' FINANCIAL SUMMARY

GOAL(S): In this exercise you will generate a Guarantors' Financial Summary report.

1. Generate the Guarantors' Financial Summary Report based on the following information:

   a. Send the report to the printer.

   b. Generate the report by account number for all accounts.

   c. Accept the default answers for the remaining fields.

   d. Compare your screen to Figure 7-1, Guarantors' Financial Summary Report Selection Screen (page 126), and press F1 to print the report.

Figure 7-1 Guarantors' Financial Summary Report Selection Screen

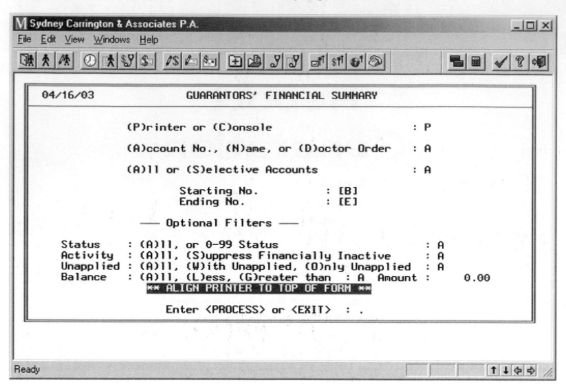

Figure 7-2 Guarantors' Financial Summary Report

```
04/16/03                      GUARANTORS' FINANCIAL SUMMARY BY ACCOUNT                      Page   1
                                Sydney Carrington & Associates P.A.
                                          All Accounts
                                          Status : All
```

Accnt #	Last Name	-Last Statement Data-	--Last Payment Data--	YTD Chgs	Unappl Cr	Pat Due AR	Balance
300	Walters,Charles	0.00	0.00	0.00	0.00	0.00	0.00
301	Rojas,Yvonne	0.00	0.00	0.00	0.00	0.00	0.00
302	Glenmore,Edward	0.00	0.00	0.00	0.00	0.00	0.00
303	Monaco,Anthony	0.00	0.00	0.00	0.00	0.00	0.00
304	Monti,Vincent	0.00	0.00	0.00	0.00	0.00	0.00
305	Viajo,Catherine	04/16/03 40.00	0.00	40.00	0.00	0.00	40.00
306	Cusack,Christine	04/16/03 98.00	0.00	98.00	0.00	0.00	98.00
307	Wyatt,John	04/16/03 73.00	0.00	73.00	0.00	0.00	73.00
308	Frost,William	04/16/03 0.00	0.00	0.00	0.00	0.00	0.00
309	Perez,Juan	04/16/03 50.00	0.00	50.00	0.00	50.00	50.00
310	Cruz,Rebecca	04/16/03 160.00	0.00	160.00	0.00	0.00	160.00
311	Vega,Roberto	04/16/03 200.00	0.00	200.00	0.00	0.00	200.00
312	Salvani,William	0.00	0.00	0.00	0.00	0.00	0.00
313	Stein,Erin	0.00	0.00	0.00	0.00	0.00	0.00
314	Fuentas,Carmen	0.00	0.00	0.00	0.00	0.00	0.00
315	Morgan,Margaret	04/16/03 126.00	0.00	126.00	0.00	0.00	126.00
316	Barker,Sharon	04/16/03 89.00	0.00	89.00	0.00	0.00	89.00
317	Lopez,Sonia	04/16/03 55.00	0.00	55.00	0.00	0.00	55.00
318	Brinkman,Gary	04/16/03 512.00	0.00	512.00	0.00	0.00	512.00
319	Miles,Wayne	04/16/03 0.00	04/16/03 123.00	123.00	0.00	0.00	0.00
320	Ramirez,Leanna	04/16/03 45.00	04/16/03 10.00	55.00	0.00	0.00	45.00
321	Marchese,Anna	04/16/03 0.00	04/16/03 40.00	40.00	0.00	0.00	0.00
322	Santos,Paul	04/16/03 131.00	04/16/03 16.00	147.00	0.00	0.00	131.00
323	Weiland,Candace	04/16/03 0.00	04/16/03 88.00	88.00	0.00	0.00	0.00
324	Hatcher,Craig	0.00	04/16/03 10.00	61.35	10.00	-10.00	-10.00
325	Roberts,Ashleigh	04/16/03 0.00	04/16/03 76.68	84.68	0.00	0.00	0.00
326	Scheller,Denise	04/16/03 15.57	04/16/03 95.43	126.00	0.00	0.00	15.57
327	Fitzpatrick,Mark	04/16/03 0.00	04/16/03 223.36	223.36	0.00	0.00	0.00
328	Penny,Robert	0.00	02/15/03 130.00	111.00	0.00	0.00	0.00
329	Knifert,John	04/16/03 63.00	04/16/03 63.00	71.00	0.00	0.00	0.00
330	Zapola,Karen	04/16/03 0.00	02/15/03 155.00	155.00	0.00	155.00	155.00
331	Jones,Elizabeth	04/16/03 60.00	02/15/03 5.00	65.00	0.00	0.00	60.00
332	Walker,Ross	0.00	0.00	0.00	0.00	0.00	0.00
333	Dwindel,Alan	0.00	0.00	0.00	0.00	0.00	0.00
334	Berntson,Allison	0.00	0.00	0.00	0.00	0.00	0.00
335	Cantorelli,Brittany	0.00	0.00	0.00	0.00	0.00	0.00
336	Valentine,Michael	0.00	0.00	0.00	0.00	0.00	0.00
337	Jermone,Pamela	0.00	04/16/03 5.00	115.00	0.00	0.00	110.00
338	Gilmore,Gerald	0.00	04/16/03 10.00	140.00	0.00	0.00	130.00
339	Stewart,Joseph	0.00	04/16/03 5.00	48.00	0.00	0.00	43.00
340	Sega,Steven	0.00	04/16/03 15.00	50.00	0.00	0.00	35.00
341	Century,Linda	0.00	04/16/03 10.00	66.00	0.00	0.00	56.00

```
          TOTALS :                                      3,172.39   10.00    195.00    2,173.57


                        ****  Number Printed : 42  ****
                        ****  Number Active  : 42  ****
```

*NOTE: **The reports will be based on the account activity entered to date. Therefore, the report information will vary by the unit exercises that have been completed.**

EXERCISE 2: CURRENT PERIOD REPORT

GOAL(S): In this exercise you will generate a Current Period Report.

1. Generate the Current Period Report based on the following information:

   a. Generate the report based on summary information.

   b. Generate the report for the period to date, for all accounts.

   c. Compare your screen to Figure 7-3, then press F1 to print the report.

Figure 7-3 Current Period Report Selection Screen

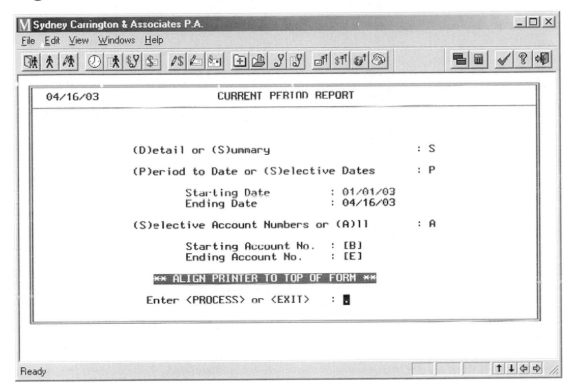

Figure 7-4 Summary Current Period Report

```
04/16/03                SUMMARY CURRENT PERIOD REPORT FOR 01/01/03 - 04/16/03           Page   1
                            Sydney Carrington & Associates P.A.
                                      All Accounts

Acct No  Name                    Phone No.         Bal Fwd  Charges  Receipts   Adjust   Balance
===============================================================================================
305      Viajo, Catherine A      (916) 694-3015              40.00                         40.00
306      Cusack, Christine G     (916) 234-1795              98.00                         98.00
307      Wyatt, John             (906) 795-2806              73.00                         73.00
308      Frost, William          (916) 326-0531              71.00               71.00      0.00
309      Perez, Juan             (917) 836-4213              50.00                         50.00
310      Cruz, Rebecca           (906) 826-9813             160.00                        160.00
311      Vega, Roberto R         (906) 845-8126             200.00                        200.00
315      Morgan, Margaret F      (907) 791-3325             126.00                        126.00
316      Barker, Sharon          (916) 331-7604              89.00                         89.00
317      Lopez, Sonia A          (917) 633-0219              55.00                         55.00
318      Brinkman, Gary          (906) 729-4819             512.00                        512.00
319      Miles, Wayne P          (906) 281-7305             123.00   123.00                 0.00
320      Ramirez, Leanna M       (907) 431-0798              55.00    10.00                45.00
321      Marchese, Anna S        (916) 698-0102              40.00    40.00                 0.00
322      Santos, Paul R          (917) 379-0834             147.00    16.00               131.00
323      Weiland, Candace        (917) 363-2963              88.00    88.00                 0.00
324      Hatcher, Craig M        (917) 795-6115              73.00    71.35    11.65      -10.00
325      Roberts, Ashleigh K     (907) 761-2315              93.00    84.68     8.32        0.00
326      Scheller, Denise L      (917) 741-1143             126.00   110.43                15.57
327      Fitzpatrick, Mark P     (906) 691-2538             243.00   223.36    19.64        0.00
328      Penny, Robert           (906) 976-2733             111.00   111.00                 0.00
329      Knifert, John           (906) 542-7893              71.00    71.00                 0.00
330      Zapola, Karen L         (906) 472-8673             155.00                        155.00
331      Jones, Elizabeth        (906) 893-2815              65.00     5.00                60.00
337      Jermone, Pamela R       (917) 923-4561             115.00     5.00               110.00
338      Gilmore, Gerald         (906) 334-2065             140.00    10.00               130.00
339      Stewart, Joseph M       (906) 245-1957              48.00     5.00                43.00
340      Sega, Steven T          (906) 796-3125              50.00    15.00                35.00
341      Century, Linda          (916) 724-6114              66.00    10.00                56.00
===============================================================================================

                 TOTALS                            0.00   3283.00   998.82   110.61    2173.57


            ****  A/R Reconciliation Not Performed - Unclosed Daily Items  ****


        ** Report Does Not Include Guarantors with ONLY Unapplied Credit Balances **
```

NOTE: The reports will be based on the account activity entered to date. Therefore, the report information will vary by the unit exercises that have been completed.

EXERCISE 3: SYSTEM FINANCIAL SUMMARY REPORT

GOAL(S): In this exercise you will generate a System Financial Summary Report.

1. Generate the System Financial Summary Report based on the following information:

   a. Select printer.

   b. Generate the report for all doctors.

   c. Show receipts and adjusts analysis.

   d. Do not skip financially inactive doctors.

   e. Compare your screen to Figure 7-5, System Financial Summary Report Selection Screen, and press F1 to print the report. Compare your printout to Figures 7-6a through 7-6c.

Figure 7-5 System Financial Summary Report Selection Screen

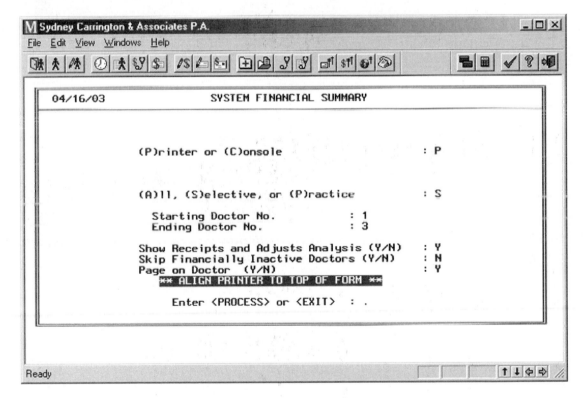

Figure 7-6a System Financial Summary – James Monroe

```
04/16/03                           SYSTEM FINANCIAL SUMMARY - DETAIL                          Page    1
                                         James T Monroe MD (1)

-------------------------------------------------------------------------------------------------------
Dates                      Charges    Receipts    Adjustments     Net A/R     Total A/R   # Proc.  Col %
-------------------------------------------------------------------------------------------------------
01/01/03 - 02/15/03         407.00      18.00        0.00          389.00      389.00        7      4.4%
01/01/03 - 02/15/03         407.00      18.00        0.00          389.00      389.00        7      4.4%
-------------------------------------------------------------------------------------------------------


                             Receipts Analysis for : James T Monroe MD (1)
-------------------------------------------------------------------------------------------------------
            Net Receipts                     PTD              YTD
-------------------------------------------------------------------------------------------------------
            Medicare                        0.00             0.00
            Insurance                       0.00             0.00
            Capitation Payments            60.00           180.00
            Patient                        18.00            18.00
            Other                           0.00             0.00
                                        -----------      -----------
            Total Receipts                 78.00           198.00
            Refunds                         0.00             0.00
                                        ============     ============
            Gross Receipts                 78.00           198.00


                             Adjustments for : James T Monroe MD (1)
-------------------------------------------------------------------------------------------------------
Adjustments          PTD          YTD       Adjustments               PTD          YTD
-------------------------------------------------------------------------------------------------------
1) General Adjustment   0.00      0.00      2) General Write-Off        0.00         0.00
3) Medicare Adjustment  0.00      0.00      4) Medicare Write-Off       0.00         0.00
5) HMO Adj & Write-Off  0.00      0.00
                    ==============  ==============
Total Adjustments       0.00      0.00


                             Refunds for : James T Monroe MD (1)
-------------------------------------------------------------------------------------------------------
Refunds              PTD          YTD       Refunds                   PTD          YTD
-------------------------------------------------------------------------------------------------------
0) Unspecified Refund   0.00      0.00      1) Incorrect Data Entry     0.00         0.00
2) Overpayment Refund   0.00      0.00      3) Returned Check           0.00         0.00
96) Acct Transfer To    0.00      0.00      97) Acct Transfer From      0.00         0.00
98) Cross-Alloc To      0.00      0.00      99) Cross-Alloc From        0.00         0.00
                    ==============  ==============
Total Refunds           0.00      0.00
```

NOTE: The reports will be based on the account activity entered to date. Therefore, the report information will vary by the unit exercises that have been completed.

Figure 7-6b System Financial Summary – Frances Simpson

SYSTEM FINANCIAL SUMMARY - DETAIL   Page   2
                                                     Frances D Simpson M.D. (2)

Dates	Charges	Receipts	Adjustments	Net A/R	Total A/R	# Proc.	Col %
01/01/03 - 02/15/03	339.00	295.00	0.00	44.00	44.00	9	87.0%
01/01/03 - 02/15/03	339.00	295.00	0.00	44.00	44.00	9	87.0%

Receipts Analysis for : Frances D Simpson M.D. (2)

Net Receipts	PTD	YTD
Medicare	0.00	0.00
Insurance	0.00	0.00
Capitation Payments	0.00	0.00
Patient	295.00	295.00
Other	0.00	0.00
Total Receipts	295.00	295.00
Refunds	0.00	0.00
Gross Receipts	295.00	295.00

Adjustments for : Frances D Simpson M.D. (2)

Adjustments	PTD	YTD	Adjustments	PTD	YTD
1) General Adjustment	0.00	0.00	2) General Write-Off	0.00	0.00
3) Medicare Adjustment	0.00	0.00	4) Medicare Write-Off	0.00	0.00
5) HMO Adj & Write-Off	0.00	0.00			
Total Adjustments	0.00	0.00			

Refunds for : Frances D Simpson M.D. (2)

Refunds	PTD	YTD	Refunds	PTD	YTD
0) Unspecified Refund	0.00	0.00	1) Incorrect Data Entry	0.00	0.00
2) Overpayment Refund	0.00	0.00	3) Returned Check	0.00	0.00
96) Acct Transfer To	0.00	0.00	97) Acct Transfer From	0.00	0.00
98) Cross-Alloc To	0.00	0.00	99) Cross-Alloc From	0.00	0.00
Total Refunds	0.00	0.00			

NOTE: The reports will be based on the account activity entered to date. Therefore, the report information will vary by the unit exercises that have been completed.

Figure 7-6c System Financial Summary – Sydney Carrington

```
04/16/03                          SYSTEM FINANCIAL SUMMARY - DETAIL                    Page    3
                                    Sydney J Carrington M.D. (3)


---------------------------------------------------------------------------------------------------
Dates                       Charges    Receipts   Adjustments      Net A/R     Total A/R  # Proc.   Col %
---------------------------------------------------------------------------------------------------
01/01/03 - 02/15/03          191.00      20.00        0.00          171.00      171.00      6        10.5%
01/01/03 - 02/15/03          191.00      20.00        0.00          171.00      171.00      6        10.5%
---------------------------------------------------------------------------------------------------



                         Receipts Analysis for : Sydney J Carrington M.D. (3)
-----------------------------------------------------------------------------------------------
              Net Receipts                  PTD            YTD
-----------------------------------------------------------------------------------------------
                 Medicare                   0.00           0.00
                 Insurance                  0.00           0.00
                 Capitation Payments      235.00         625.00
                 Patient                   20.00         437.00
                 Other                      0.00           0.00
                                        -----------    -----------
                 Total Receipts           255.00       1,062.00
                 Refunds                    0.00           0.00
                                        ===========    ===========
                 Gross Receipts           255.00       1,062.00


                          Adjustments for : Sydney J Carrington M.D. (3)
-----------------------------------------------------------------------------------------------
Adjustments              PTD          YTD     Adjustments               PTD          YTD
-----------------------------------------------------------------------------------------------
 1) General Adjustment    0.00        0.00     2) General Write-Off       0.00        0.00
 3) Medicare Adjustment   0.00        0.00     4) Medicare Write-Off      0.00        0.00
 5) HMO Adj & Write-Off   0.00        0.00
                        ==============  ==============
Total Adjustments         0.00        0.00


                            Refunds for : Sydney J Carrington M.D. (3)
-----------------------------------------------------------------------------------------------
Refunds                  PTD          YTD     Refunds                   PTD          YTD
-----------------------------------------------------------------------------------------------
 0) Unspecified Refund    0.00        0.00     1) Incorrect Data Entry    0.00        0.00
 2) Overpayment Refund    0.00        0.00     3) Returned Check          0.00        0.00
96) Acct Transfer To      0.00        0.00    97) Acct Transfer From      0.00        0.00
98) Cross-Alloc To        0.00        0.00    99) Cross-Alloc From        0.00        0.00
                        ==============  ==============
Total Refunds             0.00        0.00
```

NOTE: The reports will be based on the account activity entered to date. Therefore, the report information will vary by the unit exercises that have been completed.

EXERCISE 4: PRINTING PATIENT STATEMENTS

GOAL(S): In this exercise you will print patient statements.

1. Print patient statements based on the following information:

   a. Do not run a trial.

   b. Accept the default date.

   c. Choose the statements to be printed for all accounts in account order.

   d. Print the patient statements.

NOTE: You will generate 22 patient statements similar to Figure 7-8. Your statement for Mark Fitzpatrick may vary depending on which exercises you have completed in previous units.

Figure 7-7 Patient Statement Selection Screen

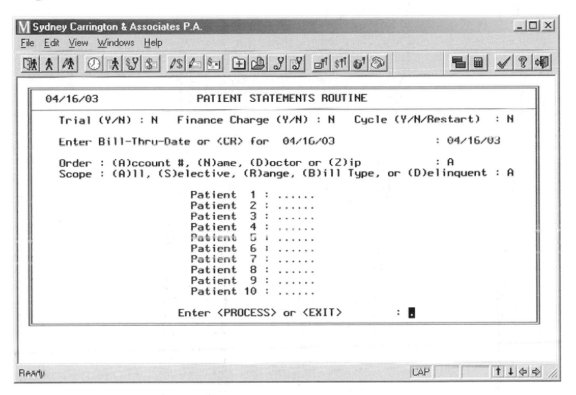

Figure 7-8 Sample Patient Statement – Mark Fitzpatrick

```
                        Sydney Carrington & Associates P.A.
                        34 Sycamore St. Suite 300
                        Madison Ca. 95653
                        (916) 398-7654


        Mark P Fitzpatrick              327          04/16/03
        1735 Parker Street
        Apt. 5A                                  Page No.   1
        Los Angeles CA 98706


   Date        Description of Transaction        Amount    Ins
   -----------------------------------------------------------------
               Balance Forward                      .00
   02/01/03    Office Estb:Comprhn               85.00      *
   02/01/03    Urinalysis                         8.00      *
   02/01/03    X-Ray Spine. Cerv (4             150.00      *
   01/10/03    Payment .... Thank Y              -2.00
   04/16/03    Payment - Pan Americ           -221.36
   04/16/03    General Write-Off                 -6.66
   04/16/03    General Write-Off                 -1.77
   04/16/03    General Write-Off                -11.21


   -----------------------------------------------------------------

                                                    .00

                       *Insurance Pending:          .00

                       Total Due From Patient :     .00


   Next Appointment :


   Aging:    CURRENT       31 - 60      61 - 90      91 - 120     121 - up

               .00           .00          .00          .00          .00

              ** Statement Due Upon Receipt * Thank You **
```

U N I T 8

Advanced Functions

In the unit exercises that follow, you will refund an overpayment, remove credit for a bad check, use Auto Pay from the insurance, rebill an insurance claim, and add a patient to a hospital rounds report. In addition, you will print an aging report and print patient data.

EXERCISE 1: REFUNDING AN OVERPAYMENT

ROBERT PENNY; ACCOUNT 328

GOAL(S): In this exercise you will correct a mistake made by the medical office during the posting procedure by refunding an overpayment.

Robert Penny was seen on 02/15/03 for an office visit with lab work. He wrote a check for the charges totaling $111. The payment was mistakenly entered as $130. The money was applied to his visit leaving a $19 unapplied credit. The account needs to be updated with a refund from the unapplied credit.

1. Based on the information above, retrieve Robert Penny's account at the Payment Entry screen and complete a refund of $19. Enter the refund as an incorrect data entry. Compare your screens to Figures 8-1 and 8-2 (page 138).

Figure 8-1 Selecting Unapplied Credit

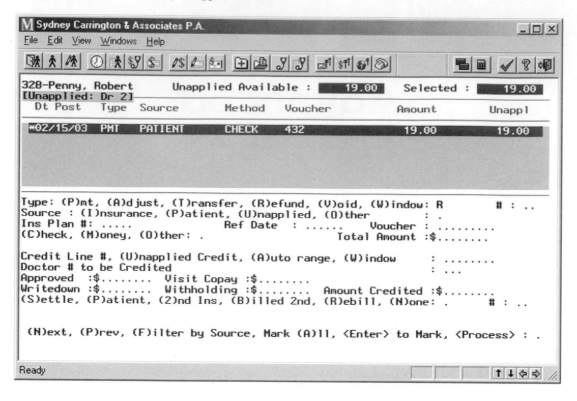

Figure 8-2 Posting a Refund

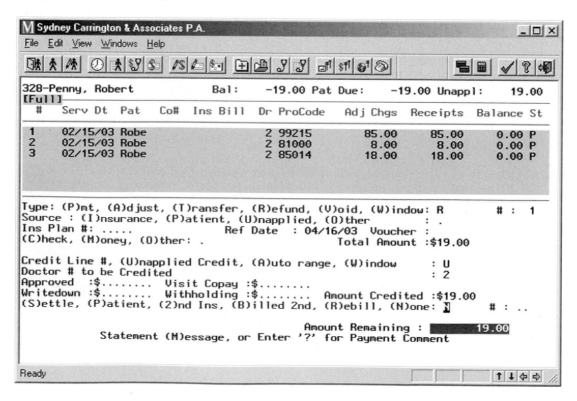

UNIT 8 Advanced Functions

EXERCISE 2: AUTO PAY WITH AN INSURANCE CHECK

JOHN KNIFERT; ACCOUNT 329

GOAL(S): In this exercise you will use the Auto Pay feature to credit an insurance check.

1. Based on the information provided from Figure 8-3, retrieve John Knifert's account and use the Auto Pay feature to post the payment. Compare your screen to Figure 8-4 (page 140) before pressing the F1 key.

Figure 8-3 Pan American Check – Knifert

```
PAN AMERICAN LIFE INSURANCE COMPANY                        623103
GROUP INSURANCE OPERATIONS  LOS ANGELES, CALIFORNIA


                                    CONTROLLER NUMBER  9087654839

                                    POLICYHOLDER NAME    WOODSIDE FD
                                    INSURED NAME         JOHN KNIFERT
                                    CLAIMANT NAME        JOHN KNIFERT
                                    DATE(S) OF SERVICE   02/15/03
PAY            SYDNEY CARRINGTON & ASSOCIATES
TO THE         34 SYCAMORE STREET
ORDER          SUITE 300                    MO. DAY YR        PAY
OF             MADISON, CALIFORNIA 95653    04 – 16 - 03      63.00

AMERICAN BANK                               BY M.K.Cist
Madison, California

⑈4011012 0000042⑈: 190151194611⑈
```

Figure 8-4 Payment Screen Before Posting

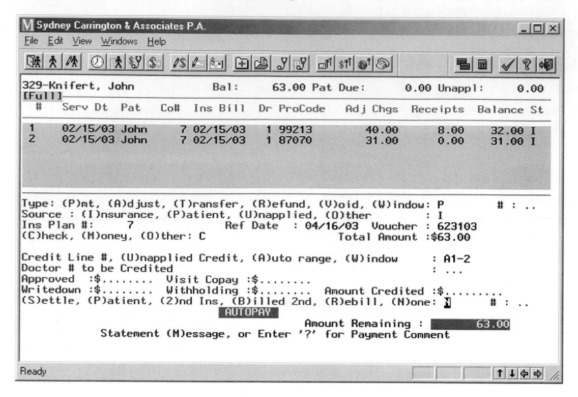

EXERCISE 3: REMOVING A BAD CHECK

KAREN ZAPOLA; ACCOUNT 330

GOAL(S): In this exercise you will remove the credit for a bad check.

The bank has returned Karen Zapola's $155 check due to nonsufficient funds. (See Figure 8-5.)

1. Post a negative payment to Karen Zapola's account to restore the item balance to unpaid. Compare your screen to Figure 8-6, then press F1.

2. Post a refund to remove the credit from the doctor's receipts. Compare your screen to Figure 8-7, then press F1.

Figure 8-5 Returned Check

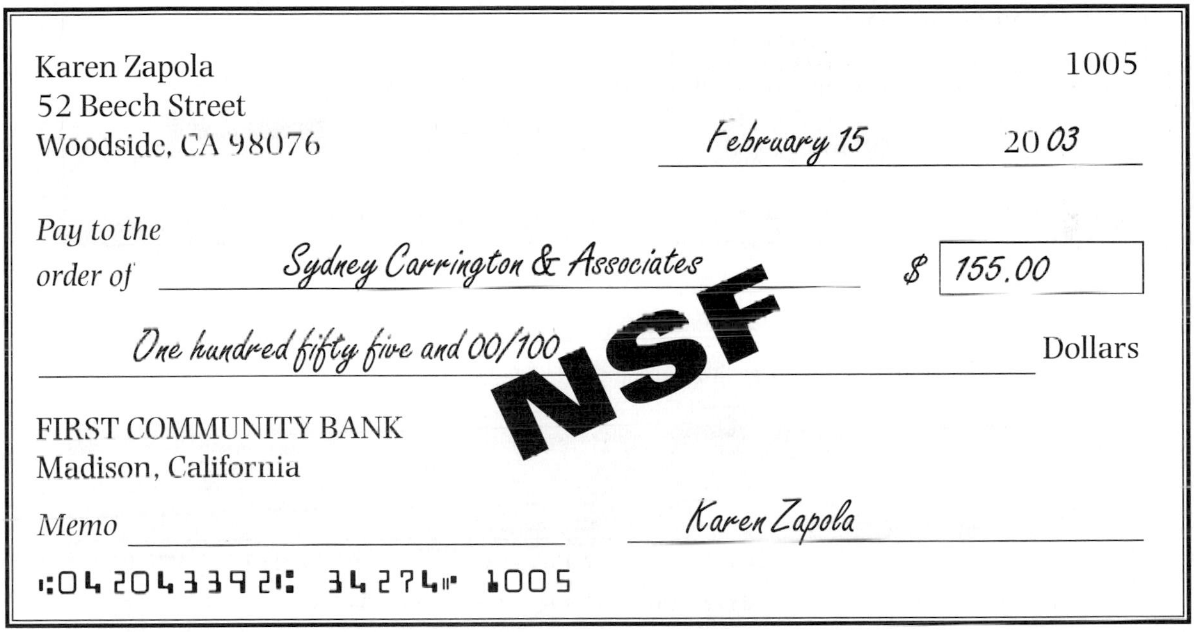

Karen Zapola   1005
52 Beech Street
Woodside, CA 98076   *February 15*   20 *03*

Pay to the
order of   *Sydney Carrington & Associates* $ | 155.00 |

        One hundred fifty five and 00/100   Dollars

FIRST COMMUNITY BANK
Madison, California

Memo   *Karen Zapola*

⑆04204339⑈ 34274⑈ 1005

Figure 8-6 Payment Screen Before Posting Reversal

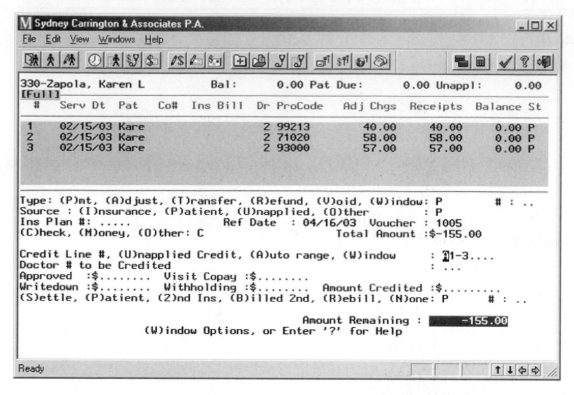

Figure 8-7 Removing the Credit Balance

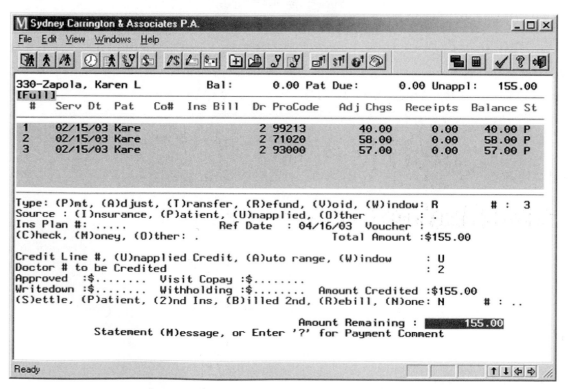

EXERCISE 4: REBILLING A LOST CLAIM

ELIZABETH JONES; ACCOUNT 331

GOAL(S): In this exercise you will rebill a lost insurance claim.

The insurance plan, Epsilon Life & Casualty, has no record of ever receiving a claim on Elizabeth Jones for her 02/15/03 visit. You must rebill the claim using an adjustment of zero dollars.

1. Using the information provided, retrieve Elizabeth Jones's account and rebill the claim that has been lost. Be sure to complete the rebill for each procedure. When you have rebilled each item, compare your screen to Figure 8-8.

Figure 8-8 After Rebill of Item – Jones

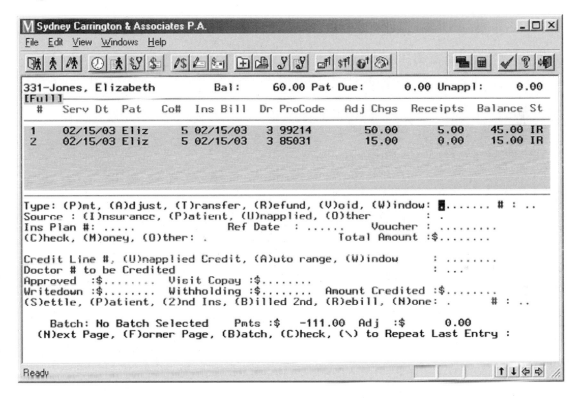

ROSS WALKER; ACCOUNT 332

GOAL(S): In this exercise you will add a patient to a hospital rounds report.

Ross Walker has been complaining of intense migraine headaches. Previous treatments have not resolved the condition. Dr. Carrington wants to admit Ross Walker to Madison General Hospital for two days and schedule an MRI and CAT scan.

1. Based on the information provided, add Ross Walker to Dr. Carrington's hospital rounds report.

    a. Have the entry appear on Dr. Carrington's rounds report. Accept the default referring doctor.

    b. Leave Room No. and Hospital Pat # blank.

2. Ross will be admitted today (04/16/03).

3. Ross' admission to the hospital is elective.

4. Compare your screen to Figure 8-9.

Figure 8-9 Hospital Rounds

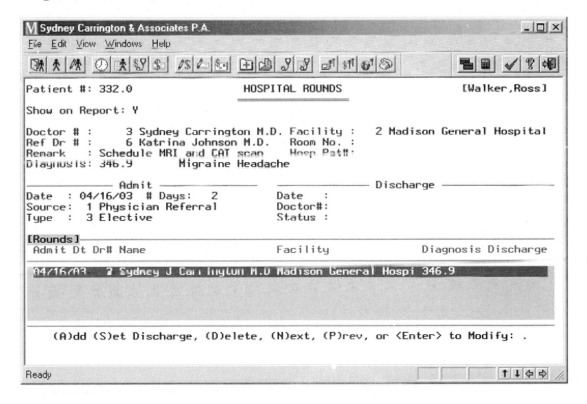

EXERCISE 6: RUNNING AGING REPORT

GOAL(S): In this exercise you will print an Aging Analysis by Practice report.

You are asked to run an aging report that compares patient and insurance due portions of accounts.

1. Print an Aging Report, selecting (A)nalysis level for the medical practice.

2. Accept the default responses for All Procedure Locations and Age by Date. Compare your screen to Figure 8-10.

NOTE: Your Aging Report may vary from Figure 8-11 depending on exercises from previous units.

Figure 8-10 Aging Report Selection Screen

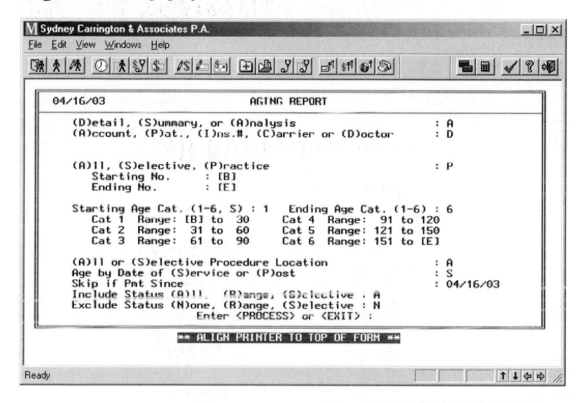

Figure 8-11 System Aging Analysis

```
04/16/03                    SYSTEM AGING ANALYSIS BY DOCTOR                    Page   1
                          Sydney Carrington & Associates P.A.
                                 SUMMARY FOR PRACTICE

                              All Procedure Locations
-------------------------------------------------------------------------------------

                   0 - 30       31 - 60       61 - 90       91 -120      121 -150      151 +
-------------------------------------------------------------------------------------

Patient   :        205.00         0.00          0.00          0.00          0.00        0.00
    %     :        100.0%         0.0%          0.0%          0.0%          0.0%        0.0%
Insurance :       1544.57        60.00          0.00          0.00          0.00        0.00
    %     :         96.3%         3.7%          0.0%          0.0%          0.0%        0.0%
-------------------------------------------------------------------------------------
Totals    :       1749.57        60.00          0.00          0.00          0.00        0.00
    %     :         96.7%         3.3%          0.0%          0.0%          0.0%        0.0%
-------------------------------------------------------------------------------------


Total Patient Receivables     :      205.00        11.3%      (Date-Patient-Responsible)
Total Insurance Receivables   :     1604.57        88.7%      (Date-Company-Billed)
Total Open Items              :     1809.57       100.0%      (Summation-of-Above)


          ****  A/R Reconciliation Not Performed - Unclosed Daily Items  ****

             ****  Report Totals Do NOT Reflect Unapplied Credits  ****
```

EXERCISE 7: PRINTING PATIENT DATA

GOAL(S): In this exercise you will print the Insurance Plan and Insured Party Information from the Display Patient Data screen.

Since Ross Walker is being admitted to the hospital you want to be familiar with his insurance coverage.

1. From the Display Patient Data screen print the hardcopies of Ross Walker's insurance coverage.

2. Since he has dual coverage be sure to position the light bar on each plan before selecting (H)ard copy. Compare your reports to Figures 8-12 and 8-13.

Figure 8-12 Guarantor Insurance Coverage

```
Patient #: 332.0            GUARANTOR INSURANCE COVERAGE              [Walker,Ross]
                        ===================================
   Policyholder: Jacqueline  Walker
   Carrier : EPSLON  Epsilon Life & Casualty      OON        : 281-65-3243
   Plan #  : 5        Epsilon Life & Casualty     Policy #   : 281653243
   Dates-From:           To :                     Other Plan

   Attn  :                                        Deductible   :    300.00
   Phone : (800) 908-7654                         Visit Copay :      0.00
   Fax   :                          Group   :
   Elig  :                          Insured: Jacqueline  Walker
   Auth  :                          User Note :



   --------------------------------------------------     --------------------

   Plan#    Plan Name                 Effective Dates    Assign  Note
   --------------------------------------------------------------------------
      5.1   Epsilon Life & Casualty           -             Y
      7.0   Pan American Health Ins.          -             Y


   --------------------------------------------------------------------------
```

Figure 8-13 Account Insurance Coverage

```
Patient #: 332              ACCOUNT INSURANCE COVERAGE               [Walker]
                     ==================================
   Policyholder: Ross M Walker
   Carrier : PANAMC  Pan American Health Ins.    SSN      : 794-85-5882
   Plan #  : 7        Pan American Health Ins.    Policy # : RP259867
   Dates-From:        To :                        Other Plan

   Attn  :                                 Deductible  :      0.00
   Phone : (213) 456-7654                  Visit Copay :      0.00
   Fax   :                        Group  : IBM
   Elig  :                        Insured: Ross M Walker
   Auth  :                        User Note :



   -------------------------------------------------------------------
   Plan#    Plan Name              Effective Dates    Assign  Note
   -------------------------------------------------------------------
     5.1   Epsilon Life & Casualty         -            Y
     7.0   Pan American Health Ins.        -            Y


   -------------------------------------------------------------------
```

EXERCISE 8: OPEN ITEMS

GOAL(S): In this exercise you will print Open Items from the Display Patient Data screen.

Since Karen Zapola's check bounced from her 02/15/03 visit, you want to print the account open items to show the detail of the credit back to the account.

1. Retrieve Karen Zapola's account at the Display Patient Data screen.

2. From Open Items, print a hard copy of each procedure on 02/15/03, showing that the check was applied and then the charges were credited back to the account.

3. Give the reports to your instructor.

EXERCISE 9: INFORMATION ON ALL CHARGES AND PAYMENTS POSTED

GOAL(S): In this exercise you will print the Financial History from the Display Patient Data screen.

1. Retrieve John Knifert's account from the Display Patient Data screen.

2. Print a hard copy of John Knifert's financial history, showing the information on all charges and payments posted.

3. Give the report to your instructor.

COMPREHENSIVE EVALUATION

The exercises that follow are intended to evaluate your understanding of **The Medical Manager** software. Complete each exercise in order, using the instructions and figures provided.

EXERCISE 1: ADD ACCOUNTS

1. Use Figures 8-14 through 8-18 (pages 156–160) to enter new patient accounts.

Figure 8-14 Patient Registration – Pamela Jermone

Patient Registration Form

Sydney Carrington & Associates
34 Sycamore Street ● Madison, CA 95653

FOR OFFICE USE ONLY	
ACCOUNT NO.:	337
DOCTOR:	#1
BILL TYPE:	11
EXTENDED INFO.:	2

TODAY'S DATE: _04/16/2003_

PATIENT INFORMATION

Jermone | Pamela | R.
PATIENT LAST NAME | FIRST NAME | MI

Self
RELATIONSHIP TO GUARANTOR

F | 01-31-72 | Single | 198-26-8878
SEX (M/F) | DATE OF BIRTH | MARITAL STATUS | SOC. SEC. #

Health Lab Corp.
EMPLOYER OR SCHOOL NAME

5 Escada Road
ADDRESS OF EMPLOYER OR SCHOOL

Madison | CA | 95653
CITY | STATE | ZIP CODE

(917) 231-5873 | Katrina Johnson, MD
EMPLOYER OR SCHOOL PHONE | REFERRED BY

E-MAIL

GUARANTOR INFORMATION

Jermone | Pamela | R. | F
RESPONSIBLE PARTY LAST NAME | FIRST NAME | MI | SEX (M/F)

P.O.Box 5673 | 49 Honey Avenue
MAILING ADDRESS | STREET ADDRESS (IF DIFFERENT)

Madison | CA | 95653
CITY | STATE | ZIP CODE

(917) 923-4561 | (917) 231-5873
(AREA CODE) HOME PHONE | (AREA CODE) WORK PHONE

01-31-72 | Single | 198-26-8878
DATE OF BIRTH | MARITAL STATUS | SOC. SEC. #

Health Lab Corp.
EMPLOYER NAME

5 Escada Road
EMPLOYER ADDRESS

Madison | CA | 95653
CITY | STATE | ZIP CODE

PRIMARY INSURANCE

Pan American Health Ins.
NAME OF PRIMARY INSURANCE COMPANY

4567 Newberry Road
ADDRESS

Los Angeles | CA | 98706
CITY | STATE | ZIP CODE

198268878 | HL
IDENTIFICATION # | GROUP NAME AND/OR #

Pamela Jermone
INSURED PERSON'S NAME (IF DIFFERENT FROM THE RESPONSIBLE PARTY)

Same
ADDRESS (IF DIFFERENT)

Same
CITY | STATE | ZIP CODE

(213) 456-7654 | 198-26-8878
PRIMARY INSURANCE PHONE NUMBER | SOC. SEC. #

Self
WHAT IS THE RESPONSIBLE PARTY'S RELATIONSHIP TO THE INSURED?

SECONDARY INSURANCE

NAME OF SECONDARY INSURANCE COMPANY

ADDRESS

CITY | STATE | ZIP CODE

IDENTIFICATION # | GROUP NAME AND/OR #

INSURED PERSON'S NAME (IF DIFFERENT FROM THE RESPONSIBLE PARTY)

ADDRESS (IF DIFFERENT)

CITY | STATE | ZIP CODE

SECONDARY INSURANCE PHONE NUMBER | SOC. SEC. #

WHAT IS THE RESPONSIBLE PARTY'S RELATIONSHIP TO THE INSURED?

I hereby consent for Sydney Carrington & Associates, P.A. to use or disclose my health information to carry out treatment, payment, and health care operations. I authorize the use of this signature on all insurance submissions. I understand that I am financially responsible for all charges whether or not paid by the insurance. I acknowledge receipt of the practice's privacy policy.

Pamela R. Jermone | 04/16/2003
PATIENT SIGNATURE | DATE

Figure 8-15 Patient Registration – Gerald Gilmore

Patient Registration Form

Sydney Carrington & Associates
34 Sycamore Street ● **Madison, CA 95653**

TODAY'S DATE: _04/16/2003_

FOR OFFICE USE ONLY

ACCOUNT NO.:	**338**
DOCTOR:	**#2**
BILL TYPE:	**11**
EXTENDED INFO.:	**2**

PATIENT INFORMATION

Gilmore	Gerald		
PATIENT LAST NAME	FIRST NAME		MI

Self
RELATIONSHIP TO GUARANTOR

M	04/07/53	Married	132-54-7713
SEX (M/F)	DATE OF BIRTH	MARITAL STATUS	SOC. SEC. #

AutoWorks
EMPLOYER OR SCHOOL NAME

13 Bellaire Avenue
ADDRESS OF EMPLOYER OR SCHOOL

Sacramento	CA	94056
CITY	STATE	ZIP CODE

(906) 271-9003	Richard Bardsley, MD
EMPLOYER OR SCHOOL PHONE	REFERRED BY

E-MAIL

GUARANTOR INFORMATION

Gilmore	Gerald		M	
RESPONSIBLE PARTY LAST NAME	FIRST NAME	MI	SEX (M/F)	

89 Galley Rd.
MAILING ADDRESS   STREET ADDRESS (IF DIFFERENT)

Sacramento	CA	94056
CITY	STATE	ZIP CODE

(906) 334-2065	(906) 271-9003
(AREA CODE) HOME PHONE	(AREA CODE) WORK PHONE

04/07/53	Married	132-54-7713
DATE OF BIRTH	MARITAL STATUS	SOC. SEC. #

AutoWorks
EMPLOYER NAME

13 Bellaire Avenue
EMPLOYER ADDRESS

Sacramento	CA	94056
CITY	STATE	ZIP CODE

PRIMARY INSURANCE

Pan American Health Ins.
NAME OF PRIMARY INSURANCE COMPANY

4567 Newberry Road
ADDRESS

Los Angeles	CA	98106
CITY	STATE	ZIP CODE

132-54-7713	AutoWorks
IDENTIFICATION #	GROUP NAME AND/OR #

Gerald Gilmore
INSURED PERSON'S NAME (IF DIFFERENT FROM THE RESPONSIBLE PARTY)

Same
ADDRESS (IF DIFFERENT)

Same		
CITY	STATE	ZIP CODE

(213) 456-7654	132-54-7713
PRIMARY INSURANCE PHONE NUMBER	SOC. SEC. #

Self
WHAT IS THE RESPONSIBLE PARTY'S RELATIONSHIP TO THE INSURED?

SECONDARY INSURANCE

NAME OF SECONDARY INSURANCE COMPANY

ADDRESS

CITY	STATE	ZIP CODE

IDENTIFICATION #	GROUP NAME AND/OR #

INSURED PERSON'S NAME (IF DIFFERENT FROM THE RESPONSIBLE PARTY)

ADDRESS (IF DIFFERENT)

CITY	STATE	ZIP CODE

SECONDARY INSURANCE PHONE NUMBER	SOC. SEC. #

WHAT IS THE RESPONSIBLE PARTY'S RELATIONSHIP TO THE INSURED?

I hereby consent for Sydney Carrington & Associates, P.A. to use or disclose my health information to carry out treatment, payment, and health care operations. I authorize the use of this signature on all insurance submissions. I understand that I am financially responsible for all charges whether or not paid by the insurance. I acknowledge receipt of the practice's privacy policy.

Gerald Gilmore	04/16/2003
PATIENT SIGNATURE	DATE

Figure 8-16 Patient Registration – Joseph Stewart

Patient Registration Form

Sydney Carrington & Associates
34 Sycamore Street • Madison, CA 95653

TODAY'S DATE: _04/16/2003_

FOR OFFICE USE ONLY	
ACCOUNT NO.:	**339**
DOCTOR:	**#3**
BILL TYPE:	**11**
EXTENDED INFO.:	**2**

PATIENT INFORMATION

Stewart *Joseph* *M*
PATIENT LAST NAME FIRST NAME MI

Self
RELATIONSHIP TO GUARANTOR

M | *01-19-40* | *Married* | *144-36-7861*
SEX (M/F) DATE OF BIRTH MARITAL STATUS SOC. SEC. #

NP Penske, Inc.
EMPLOYER OR SCHOOL NAME

173 Marland Court
ADDRESS OF EMPLOYER OR SCHOOL

Floral City | *CA* | *94064*
CITY STATE ZIP CODE

(917) 381-5467 | *Jason Detrasnik, MD*
EMPLOYER OR SCHOOL PHONE REFERRED BY

E-MAIL

GUARANTOR INFORMATION

Stewart *Joseph* *M* | *M*
RESPONSIBLE PARTY LAST NAME FIRST NAME MI SEX (M/F)

600 Pyramid Avenue – Apt. 847
MAILING ADDRESS STREET ADDRESS (IF DIFFERENT)

Woodside | *CA* | *98076*
CITY STATE ZIP CODE

(906) 795-2542 | *(917) 381-5467*
(AREA CODE) HOME PHONE (AREA CODE) WORK PHONE

01-19-40 | *Married* | *144-36-7861*
DATE OF BIRTH MARITAL STATUS SOC. SEC. #

NP Penske, Inc.
EMPLOYER NAME

173 Marland Court
EMPLOYER ADDRESS

Floral City | *CA* | *94064*
CITY STATE ZIP CODE

PRIMARY INSURANCE

Pan American Health Ins.
NAME OF PRIMARY INSURANCE COMPANY

4567 Newberry Road
ADDRESS

Los Angeles | *CA* | *98706*
CITY STATE ZIP CODE

144-36-7861 | *NP*
IDENTIFICATION # GROUP NAME AND/OR #

Joseph Stewart
INSURED PERSON'S NAME (IF DIFFERENT FROM THE RESPONSIBLE PARTY)

Same
ADDRESS (IF DIFFERENT)

Same
CITY STATE ZIP CODE

(213) 456-7654 | *144-36-7861*
PRIMARY INSURANCE PHONE NUMBER SOC. SEC. #

Self
WHAT IS THE RESPONSIBLE PARTY'S RELATIONSHIP TO THE INSURED?

SECONDARY INSURANCE

NAME OF SECONDARY INSURANCE COMPANY

ADDRESS

CITY STATE ZIP CODE

IDENTIFICATION # GROUP NAME AND/OR #

INSURED PERSON'S NAME (IF DIFFERENT FROM THE RESPONSIBLE PARTY)

ADDRESS (IF DIFFERENT)

CITY STATE ZIP CODE

SECONDARY INSURANCE PHONE NUMBER SOC. SEC. #

WHAT IS THE RESPONSIBLE PARTY'S RELATIONSHIP TO THE INSURED?

I hereby consent for Sydney Carrington & Associates, P.A. to use or disclose my health information to carry out treatment, payment, and health care operations. I authorize the use of this signature on all insurance submissions. I understand that I am financially responsible for all charges whether or not paid by the insurance. I acknowledge receipt of the practice's privacy policy.

Joseph Stewart _04/16/2003_
PATIENT SIGNATURE DATE

Figure 8-17 Patient Registration – Steven Sega

Patient Registration Form

Sydney Carrington & Associates
34 Sycamore Street ● Madison, CA 95653

TODAY'S DATE: _04/16/2003_

FOR OFFICE USE ONLY	
ACCOUNT NO.:	**340**
DOCTOR:	**#1**
BILL TYPE:	**11**
EXTENDED INFO.:	

PATIENT INFORMATION

Sega	_Steven_	_T_
PATIENT LAST NAME	FIRST NAME	MI

Self
RELATIONSHIP TO GUARANTOR

_M_	_12-02-55_	_Married_	_013-25-7614_
SEX (M/F)	DATE OF BIRTH	MARITAL STATUS	SOC. SEC. #

Home Front Realty
EMPLOYER OR SCHOOL NAME

544 Beach Comb Lane
ADDRESS OF EMPLOYER OR SCHOOL

Woodside	_CA_	_98076_
CITY	STATE	ZIP CODE

_(917) 287-1445_	_James Johnson, MD_
EMPLOYER OR SCHOOL PHONE	REFERRED BY

E-MAIL

GUARANTOR INFORMATION

Sega	_Steven_	_T_	_M_
RESPONSIBLE PARTY LAST NAME	FIRST NAME	MI	SEX (M/F)

2536 Franklin Street	
MAILING ADDRESS	STREET ADDRESS (IF DIFFERENT)

Floral City	_CA_	_94064_
CITY	STATE	ZIP CODE

_(906) 796-3125_	_(917) 287-1445_
(AREA CODE) HOME PHONE	(AREA CODE) WORK PHONE

_12-02-55_	_Married_	_013-25-7614_
DATE OF BIRTH	MARITAL STATUS	SOC. SEC. #

Home Front Realty
EMPLOYER NAME

544 Beach Comb Lane
EMPLOYER ADDRESS

Woodside	_CA_	_98076_
CITY	STATE	ZIP CODE

PRIMARY INSURANCE

Pan American Health Ins.
NAME OF PRIMARY INSURANCE COMPANY

4567 Newberry Road
ADDRESS

Los Angeles	_CA_	_98706_
CITY	STATE	ZIP CODE

_141 11 315_	
IDENTIFICATION #	GROUP NAME AND/OR #

Rachel Sega
INSURED PERSON'S NAME (IF DIFFERENT FROM THE RESPONSIBLE PARTY)

Same
ADDRESS (IF DIFFERENT)

Same		
CITY	STATE	ZIP CODE

_(213) 456-7654_	_141-11-315_
PRIMARY INSURANCE PHONE NUMBER	SOC. SEC. #

Husband
WHAT IS THE RESPONSIBLE PARTY'S RELATIONSHIP TO THE INSURED?

SECONDARY INSURANCE

Epsilon Life and Casualty
NAME OF SECONDARY INSURANCE COMPANY

P.O. Box 189
ADDRESS

Macon	_CA_	_31298_
CITY	STATE	ZIP CODE

_013257614_	
IDENTIFICATION #	GROUP NAME AND/OR #

Steven Sega
INSURED PERSON'S NAME (IF DIFFERENT FROM THE RESPONSIBLE PARTY)

Same
ADDRESS (IF DIFFERENT)

Same		
CITY	STATE	ZIP CODE

_(800) 908-7654_	_013-25-7614_
SECONDARY INSURANCE PHONE NUMBER	SOC. SEC. #

Self
WHAT IS THE RESPONSIBLE PARTY'S RELATIONSHIP TO THE INSURED?

I hereby consent for Sydney Carrington & Associates, P.A. to use or disclose my health information to carry out treatment, payment, and health care operations. I authorize the use of this signature on all insurance submissions. I understand that I am financially responsible for all charges whether or not paid by the insurance. I acknowledge receipt of the practice's privacy policy.

Steven Sega	_04/16/2003_
PATIENT SIGNATURE	DATE

Figure 8-18 Patient Registration – Linda Century

Patient Registration Form

Sydney Carrington & Associates
34 Sycamore Street ● Madison, CA 95653

TODAY'S DATE: _04/16/03_

FOR OFFICE USE ONLY	
ACCOUNT NO.:	**341**
DOCTOR:	**#2**
BILL TYPE:	**11**
EXTENDED INFO.:	**2**

PATIENT INFORMATION

Century | _Linda_
PATIENT LAST NAME | FIRST NAME | MI

Self
RELATIONSHIP TO GUARANTOR

_F_ | _02-27-63_ | _Married_ | _136-45-2536_
SEX (M/F) | DATE OF BIRTH | MARITAL STATUS | SOC. SEC. #

Bell Sound, Corp.
EMPLOYER OR SCHOOL NAME

8 Kranton Street
ADDRESS OF EMPLOYER OR SCHOOL

Los Angeles | _CA_ | _98706_
CITY | STATE | ZIP CODE

_(916) 474-2536_ | _Guy Shelton, MD_
EMPLOYER OR SCHOOL PHONE | REFERRED BY

E-MAIL

GUARANTOR INFORMATION

Century | _Linda_ | | _F_
RESPONSIBLE PARTY LAST NAME | FIRST NAME | MI | SEX (M/F)

14 Candle Lane
MAILING ADDRESS | STREET ADDRESS (IF DIFFERENT)

Los Angeles | _CA_ | _98706_
CITY | STATE | ZIP CODE

_(916) 724-6114_ | _(916) 474-2536_
(AREA CODE) HOME PHONE | (AREA CODE) WORK PHONE

_02-27-63_ | _Married_ | _136-45-2536_
DATE OF BIRTH | MARITAL STATUS | SOC. SEC. #

Bell Sound, Corp.
EMPLOYER NAME

8 Kranton Street
EMPLOYER ADDRESS

Los Angeles | _CA_ | _98706_
CITY | STATE | ZIP CODE

PRIMARY INSURANCE

Pan American Health Ins.
NAME OF PRIMARY INSURANCE COMPANY

4567 Newberry Road
ADDRESS

Los Angeles | _CA_ | _98706_
CITY | STATE | ZIP CODE

_471-66-2317_
IDENTIFICATION # | GROUP NAME AND/OR #

Robert Century
INSURED PERSON'S NAME (IF DIFFERENT FROM THE RESPONSIBLE PARTY)

Same
ADDRESS (IF DIFFERENT)

Same
CITY | STATE | ZIP CODE

_(213) 456-7654_ | _471-66-2317_
PRIMARY INSURANCE PHONE NUMBER | SOC. SEC. #

Wife
WHAT IS THE RESPONSIBLE PARTY'S RELATIONSHIP TO THE INSURED?

SECONDARY INSURANCE

NAME OF SECONDARY INSURANCE COMPANY

ADDRESS

CITY | STATE | ZIP CODE

IDENTIFICATION # | GROUP NAME AND/OR #

INSURED PERSON'S NAME (IF DIFFERENT FROM THE RESPONSIBLE PARTY)

ADDRESS (IF DIFFERENT)

CITY | STATE | ZIP CODE

SECONDARY INSURANCE PHONE NUMBER | SOC. SEC. #

WHAT IS THE RESPONSIBLE PARTY'S RELATIONSHIP TO THE INSURED?

I hereby consent for Sydney Carrington & Associates, P.A. to use or disclose my health information to carry out treatment, payment, and health care operations. I authorize the use of this signature on all insurance submissions. I understand that I am financially responsible for all charges whether or not paid by the insurance. I acknowledge receipt of the practice's privacy policy.

Linda Century | _04/16/03_
PATIENT SIGNATURE | DATE

EXERCISE 2: POST PROCEDURES AND COPAYMENTS FROM THE PROCEDURE ENTRY SCREEN AND SCHEDULE FOLLOW-UP APPOINTMENTS

1. Use Figures 8-19 through 8-23 (pages 162–166) to post procedures to patient accounts. Be sure to look at the Amount Paid portion of the encounter forms to determine the copayment paid. Continue to the Appointment screen and schedule the follow-up appointment.

Figure 8-19 Encounter Form – Gerald Gilmore

Sydney Carrington & Associates P.A.
34 Sycamore Street   Suite 300
Madison, CA 95653

Date: 04/16/2003

Voucher No.:   1031

Time:

Patient: Gerald Gilmore
Guarantor:

Patient No: 338.0

Doctor: 2 - F. Simpson

	CPT	DESCRIPTION	FEE
	OFFICE/HOSPITAL CONSULTS		
☐	99201	Office New:Focused Hx-Exam	
☐	99202	Office New:Expanded Hx-Exam	
☒	99211	Office Estb:Min/None Hx-Exa	$25
☐	99212	Office Estb:Focused Hx-Exam	
☐	99213	Office Estb:Expanded Hx-Exa	
☐	99214	Office Estb:Detailed Hx-Exa	
☐	99215	Office Estb:Comprhn Hx-Exam	
☐	99221	Hosp. Initial:Comprh Hx-	
☐	99223	Hosp.Ini:Comprh Hx-Exam/Hi	
☐	99231	Hosp. Subsequent: S-Fwd	
☐	99232	Hosp. Subsequent: Comprhn Hx	
☐	99233	Hosp. Subsequent: Ex/Hi	
☐	99238	Hospital Visit Discharge Ex	
☐	99371	Telephone Consult - Simple	
☐	99372	Telephone Consult - Intermed	
☐	99373	Telephone Consult - Complex	
☐	90843	Counseling - 25 minutes	
☐	90844	Counseling - 50 minutes	
☐	90865	Counseling - Special Interview	
	IMMUNIZATIONS/INJECTIONS		
☐	90585	BCG Vaccine	
☐	90659	Influenza Virus Vaccine	
☐	90701	Immunization-DTP	
☐	90702	DT Vaccine	
☐	90703	Tetanus Toxoids	
☐	90732	Pneumococcal Vaccine	
☐	90746	Hepatitis B Vaccine	
☐	90749	Immunization; Unlisted	

	CPT	DESCRIPTION	FEE
	LABORATORY/RADIOLOGY		
☐	81000	Urinalysis	
☐	81002	Urinalysis; Pregnancy Test	
☐	82951	Glucose Tolerance Test	
☐	84478	Triglycerides	
☐	84550	Uric Acid: Blood Chemistry	
☐	84830	Ovulation Test	
☐	85014	Hematocrit	
☐	85031	Hemogram, Complete Blood Wk	
☐	86403	Particle Agglutination Test	
☐	86485	Skin Test; Candida	
☐	86580	TB Intradermal Test	
☐	86585	TB Tine Test	
☐	87070	Culture	
☐	70190	X-Ray; Optic Foramina	
☐	70210	X-Ray Sinuses Complete	
☐	71010	Radiological Exam Ent Spine	
☒	71020	X-Ray Chest Pa & Lat	$58
☐	72050	X-Ray Spine, Cerv (4 views)	
☐	72090	X-Ray Spine; Scoliosis Ex	
☐	72110	Spine, lumbosacral; a/p & Lat	
☐	73030	Shoulder-Comp, min w/ 2vws	
☐	73070	Elbow, anteropost & later vws	
☐	73120	X-Ray; Hand, 2 views	
☐	73560	X-Ray, Knee, 1 or 2 views	
☐	74022	X-Ray; Abdomen, Complete	
☐	75552	Cardiac Magnetic Res Img	
☐	76020	X-Ray; Bone Age Studies	
☐	76088	Mammary Ductogram Complete	
☐	78465	Myocardial Perfusion Img	

	CPT	DESCRIPTION	FEE
	PROCEDURES/TESTS		
☐	00452	Anesthesia for Rad Surgery	
☐	11100	Skin Biopsy	
☐	15852	Dressing Change	
☐	29075	Cast Appl. - Lower Arm	
☐	29530	Strapping of Knee	
☐	29705	Removal/Revis of Cast w/Exa	
☐	53670	Catheterization Incl. Suppl	
☐	57452	Colposcopy	
☐	57505	ECC	
☐	69420	Myringotomy	
☐	92081	Visual Field Examination	
☐	92100	Serial Tonometry Exam	
☐	92120	Tonography	
☐	92552	Pure Tone Audiometry	
☐	92567	Tympanometry	
☒	93000	Electrocardiogram	$57
☐	93015	Exercise Stress Test (ETT)	
☐	93017	ETT Tracing Only	
☐	93040	Electrocardiogram - Rhythm	
☐	96100	Psychological Testing	
☐	99000	Specimen Handling	
☐	99058	Office Emergency Care	
☐	99070	Surgical Tray - Misc.	
☐	99080	Special Reports of Med Rec	
☐	99195	Phlebotomy	
☐			
☐			
☐			

	ICD-9 CODE DIAGNOSIS	
☐	009.0	Ill-defined Intestinal Infect
☐	133.2	Establish Baseline
☐	174.9	Breast Cancer
☐	185.0	Prostate Cancer
☐	250	Diabetes Mellitus
☐	272.4	Hyperlipidemia
☐	282.5	Anemia - Sickle Trait
☐	282.60	Anemia - Sickle Cell
☐	285.9	Anemia, Unspecified
☐	300.4	Neurotic Depression
☐	340	Multiple Sclerosis
☐	342.9	Hemiplegia - Unspecified
☐	346.9	Migraine Headache
☐	352.9	Cranial Neuralgia
☐	354.0	Carpal Tunnel Syndrome
☐	355.0	Sciatic Nerve Root Lesion
☐	366.9	Cataract
☐	386.0	Vertigo
☐	401.1	Essential Hypertension
☐	414.9	Ischemic Hearth Disease
☐	428.0	Congestive Heart Failure

	ICD-9 CODE DIAGNOSIS	
☐	435.0	Basilar Artery Syndrome
☐	440.0	Atherosclerosis
☐	442.81	Carotid Artery
☐	460.0	Common Cold
☐	461.9	Acute Sinusitis
☐	474.0	Tonsillitis
☐	477.9	Hay Fever
☒	487.0	Flu
☐	496	Chronic Airway Obstruction
☐	522	Low Red Blood Count
☐	524.6	Temporo-Mandibular Jnt Synd
☐	538.8	Stomach Pain
☐	553.3	Hiatal Hernia
☐	564.1	Spastic Colon
☐	571.4	Chronic Hepatitis
☐	571.5	Cirrhosis of Liver
☐	573.3	Hepatitis
☐	575.2	Obstruction of Gallbladder
☐	648.2	Anemia - Compl. Pregnancy
☐	715.90	Osteoarthritis - Unspec
☐	721.3	Lumbar Osteo/Spondylarthrit

	ICD-9 CODE DIAGNOSIS	
☐	724.2	Pain: Lower Back
☐	727.6	Rupture of Achilles Tendon
☐	780.1	Hallucinations
☐	780.3	Convulsions
☐	780.5	Sleep Disturbances
☐	783.0	Anorexia
☐	783.1	Abnormal Weight Gain
☐	783.2	Abnormal Weight Loss
☐	830.6	Dislocated Hip
☐	830.9	Dislocated Shoulder
☐	841.2	Sprained Wrist
☐	842.5	Sprained Ankle
☐	891.2	Fractured Tibia
☐	892.0	Fractured Fibula
☐	919.5	Insect Bite, Nonvenomous
☐	921.1	Contus Eyelid/Perioc Area
☐	v16.3	Fam. Hist of Breast Cancer
☐	v17.4	Fam. Hist of Cardiovasc Dis
☐	v20.2	Well Child
☐	v22.0	Pregnancy - First Normal
☐	v22.1	Pregnancy - Normal

Previous Balance	Today's Charges	Total Due	Amount Paid	New Balance
			$10 check #623	

I hereby authorize release of any information acquired in the course of examination or treatment and allow a photocopy of my signature to be used.

Follow Up

PRN _____ Weeks _____   Months _____   Units _____

Next Appointment Date: April 25   Time: 1:15   Follow-up

Recheck

Figure 8-20 Encounter Form – Steven Sega

Sydney Carrington & Associates P.A.
34 Sycamore Street   Suite 300
Madison, CA 95653

Date: 04/16/2003   Voucher No.: 1032

Time:

Patient: Steven Sega   Patient No: 340.0
Guarantor: Doctor: 1 - J. Monroe

	CPT	DESCRIPTION	FEE
	OFFICE/HOSPITAL CONSULTS		
☐	99201	Office New:Focused Hx-Exam	
☐	99202	Office New:Expanded Hx-Exam	
☐	99211	Office Estb:Min/None Hx-Exa	
☐	99212	Office Estb:Focused Hx-Exam	
☐	99213	Office Estb:Expanded Hx-Exa	
☒	99214	Office Estb:Detailed Hx-Exa	$50
☐	99215	Office Estb:Comprhn Hx-Exam	
☐	99221	Hosp. Initial:Comprh Hx-	
☐	99223	Hosp.Ini:Comprh Hx-Exam/Hi	
☐	99231	Hosp. Subsequent: S-Fwd	
☐	99232	Hosp. Subsequent: Comprhn Hx	
☐	99233	Hosp. Subsequent: Ex/Hi	
☐	99200	Hospital Visit Discharge Ex	
☐	99371	Telephone Consult - Simple	
☐	99372	Telephone Consult - Intermed	
☐	99373	Telephone Consult - Complex	
☐	90843	Counseling - 25 minutes	
☐	90844	Counseling - 50 minutes	
☐	90865	Counseling - Special Interview	
	IMMUNIZATIONS/INJECTIONS		
☐	90585	BCG Vaccine	
☐	90659	Influenza Virus Vaccine	
☐	90701	Immunization-DTP	
☐	90702	DT Vaccine	
☐	90703	Tetanus Toxoids	
☐	90732	Pneumococcal Vaccine	
☐	90746	Hepatitis B Vaccine	
☐	90749	Immunization; Unlisted	

	CPT	DESCRIPTION	FEE
	LABORATORY/RADIOLOGY		
☐	81000	Urinalysis	
☐	81002	Urinalysis; Pregnancy Test	
☐	82951	Glucose Tolerance Test	
☐	84478	Triglycerides	
☐	84550	Uric Acid: Blood Chemistry	
☐	84830	Ovulation Test	
☐	85014	Hematocrit	
☐	85031	Hemogram, Complete Blood Wk	
☐	86403	Particle Agglutination Test	
☐	86485	Skin Test; Candida	
☐	86580	TB Intradermal Test	
☐	86585	TB Tine Test	
☐	87070	Culture	
☐	70190	X-Ray; Optic Foramina	
☐	70210	X-Ray Sinuses Complete	
☐	71010	Radiological Exam Ent Spine	
☐	71020	X-Ray Chest Pa & Lat	
☐	72050	X-Ray Spine, Cerv (4 views)	
☐	72090	X-Ray Spine; Scoliosis Ex	
☐	72110	Spine, lumbosacral; a/p & Lat	
☐	73030	Shoulder-Comp, min w/ 2vws	
☐	73070	Elbow, anteropost & later vws	
☐	73120	X-Ray: Hand. 2 views	
☐	73560	X-Ray, Knee, 1 or 2 views	
☐	74022	X-Ray; Abdomen, Complete	
☐	75552	Cardiac Magnetic Res Img	
☐	76020	X-Ray; Bone Age Studies	
☐	76088	Mammary Ductogram Complete	
☐	78465	Myocardial Perfusion Img	

	CPT	DESCRIPTION	FEE
	PROCEDURES/TESTS		
☐	00452	Anesthesia for Rad Surgery	
☐	11100	Skin Biopsy	
☐	15852	Dressing Change	
☐	29075	Cast Appl. - Lower Arm	
☐	29530	Strapping of Knee	
☐	29705	Removal/Revis of Cast w/Exa	
☐	53670	Catheterization Incl. Suppl	
☐	57452	Colposcopy	
☐	57505	ECC	
☐	69420	Myringotomy	
☐	92081	Visual Field Examination	
☐	92100	Serial Tonometry Exam	
☐	92120	Tonography	
☐	92552	Pure Tone Audiometry	
☐	92567	Tympanometry	
☐	93000	Electrocardiogram	
☐	93015	Exercise Stress Test (ETT)	
☐	93017	ETT Tracing Only	
☐	93040	Electrocardiogram - Rhythm	
☐	96100	Psychological Testing	
☐	99000	Specimen Handling	
☐	99058	Office Emergency Care	
☐	99070	Surgical Tray - Misc.	
☐	99080	Special Reports of Med Rec	
☐	99195	Phlebotomy	
☐		_____	
☐		_____	
☐		_____	
☐		_____	

	ICD-9 CODE DIAGNOSIS	
☐	009.0	Ill-defined Intestinal Infect
☐	133.2	Establish Baseline
☐	174.9	Breast Cancer
☐	185.0	Prostate Cancer
☐	250	Diabetes Mellitus
☐	272.4	Hyperlipidemia
☐	282.5	Anemia - Sickle Trait
☐	282.60	Anemia - Sickle Cell
☐	285.9	Anemia, Unspecified
☐	300.4	Neurotic Depression
☐	340	Multiple Sclerosis
☐	342.9	Hemiplegia - Unspecified
☐	346.9	Migraine Headache
☐	352.9	Cranial Neuralgia
☐	354.0	Carpal Tunnel Syndrome
☐	355.0	Sciatic Nerve Root Lesion
☐	366.9	Cataract
☐	386.0	Vertigo
☐	401.1	Essential Hypertension
☐	414.9	Ischemic Hearth Disease
☐	428.0	Congestive Heart Failure

	ICD-9 CODE DIAGNOSIS	
☐	435.0	Basilar Artery Syndrome
☐	440.0	Atherosclerosis
☐	442.81	Carotid Artery
☐	460.0	Common Cold
☐	461.9	Acute Sinusitis
☐	474.0	Tonsillitis
☐	477.9	Hay Fever
☐	487.0	Flu
☐	496	Chronic Airway Obstruction
☐	522	Low Red Blood Count
☐	524.6	Temporo-Mandibular Jnt Synd
☐	538.8	Stomach Pain
☐	553.3	Hiatal Hernia
☒	564.1	Spastic Colon
☐	571.4	Chronic Hepatitis
☐	571.5	Cirrhosis of Liver
☐	573.3	Hepatitis
☐	575.2	Obstruction of Gallbladder
☐	648.2	Anemia - Compl. Pregnancy
☐	715.90	Osteoarthritis - Unspec
☐	721.3	Lumbar Osteo/Spondylarthrit

	ICD-9 CODE DIAGNOSIS	
☐	724.2	Pain: Lower Back
☐	727.6	Rupture of Achilles Tendon
☐	780.1	Hallucinations
☐	780.3	Convulsions
☐	780.5	Sleep Disturbances
☐	783.0	Anorexia
☐	783.1	Abnormal Weight Gain
☐	783.2	Abnormal Weight Loss
☐	830.6	Dislocated Hip
☐	830.9	Dislocated Shoulder
☐	841.2	Sprained Wrist
☐	842.5	Sprained Ankle
☐	891.2	Fractured Tibia
☐	892.0	Fractured Fibula
☐	919.5	Insect Bite, Nonvenomous
☐	921.1	Contus Eyelid/Perioc Area
☐	v16.3	Fam. Hist of Breast Cancer
☐	v17.4	Fam. Hist of Cardiovasc Dis
☐	v20.2	Well Child
☐	v22.0	Pregnancy - First Normal
☐	v22.1	Pregnancy - Normal

Previous Balance	Today's Charges	Total Due	Amount Paid	New Balance
_____	_____	_____	$15 check #112	

Follow Up

PRN _____ Weeks _____   Months _____ Units _____

Next Appointment Date: April 18   Time: 4:00 Personal consult
                                                        30 minutes

I hereby authorize release of any information acquired in the course of examination or treatment and allow a photocopy of my signature to be used.

_____

Figure 8-21 Encounter Form – Linda Century

Sydney Carrington & Associates P.A.
34 Sycamore Street   Suite 300
Madison, CA 95653

Date: 04/16/2003

Time:

Patient: Linda Century
Guarantor:

Voucher No.: 1033

Patient No: 341.0
Doctor: 2 - F. Simpson

CPT	DESCRIPTION	FEE
OFFICE/HOSPITAL CONSULTS		
☐ 99201	Office New:Focused Hx-Exam	
☐ 99202	Office New:Expanded Hx-Exam	
☐ 99211	Office Estb:Min/None Hx-Exa	
☐ 99212	Office Estb:Focused Hx-Exam	
☒ 99213	Office Estb:Expanded Hx-Exa	$40
☐ 99214	Office Estb:Detailed Hx-Exa	
☐ 99215	Office Estb:Comprhn Hx-Exam	
☐ 99221	Hosp. Initial:Comprh Hx-	
☐ 99223	Hosp.Ini:Comprh Hx-Exam/Hi	
☐ 99231	Hosp. Subsequent: S-Fwd	
☐ 99232	Hosp. Subsequent: Comprhn Hx	
☐ 99233	Hosp. Subsequent: Ex/Hi	
☐ 99238	Hospital Visit Discharge Ex	
☐ 99371	Telephone Consult - Simple	
☐ 99372	Telephone Consult - Intermed	
☐ 99373	Telephone Consult - Complex	
☐ 90843	Counseling - 25 minutes	
☐ 90844	Counseling - 50 minutes	
☐ 90865	Counseling - Special Interview	
IMMUNIZATIONS/INJECTIONS		
☐ 90585	BCG Vaccine	
☐ 90659	Influenza Virus Vaccine	
☐ 90701	Immunization-DTP	
☐ 90702	DT Vaccine	
☐ 90703	Tetanus Toxoids	
☐ 90732	Pneumococcal Vaccine	
☐ 90746	Hepatitis B Vaccine	
☐ 90749	Immunization; Unlisted	

CPT	DESCRIPTION	FEE
LABORATORY/RADIOLOGY		
☒ 81000	Urinalysis	$8
☐ 81002	Urinalysis; Pregnancy Test	
☐ 82951	Glucose Tolerance Test	
☐ 84478	Triglycerides	
☐ 84550	Uric Acid: Blood Chemistry	
☐ 84830	Ovulation Test	
☒ 85014	Hematocrit	$18
☐ 85031	Hemogram, Complete Blood Wk	
☐ 86403	Particle Agglutination Test	
☐ 86485	Skin Test; Candida	
☐ 86580	TB Intradermal Test	
☐ 86585	TB Tine Test	
☐ 87070	Culture	
☐ 70190	X-Ray; Optic Foramina	
☐ 70210	X-Ray Sinuses Complete	
☐ 71010	Radiological Exam Ent Spine	
☐ 71020	X-Ray Chest Pa & Lat	
☐ 72050	X-Ray Spine, Cerv (4 views)	
☐ 72090	X-Ray Spine; Scoliosis Ex	
☐ 72110	Spine, lumbosacral; a/p & Lat	
☐ 73030	Shoulder-Comp, min w/ 2vws	
☐ 73070	Elbow, anteropost & later vws	
☐ 73120	X-Ray; Hand, 2 views	
☐ 73560	X-Ray, Knee, 1 or 2 views	
☐ 74022	X-Ray; Abdomen, Complete	
☐ 75552	Cardiac Magnetic Res Img	
☐ 76020	X-Ray; Bone Age Studies	
☐ 76088	Mammary Ductogram Complete	
☐ 78465	Myocardial Perfusion Img	

CPT	DESCRIPTION	FEE
PROCEDURES/TESTS		
☐ 00452	Anesthesia for Rad Surgery	
☐ 11100	Skin Biopsy	
☐ 15852	Dressing Change	
☐ 29075	Cast Appl. - Lower Arm	
☐ 29530	Strapping of Knee	
☐ 29705	Removal/Revis of Cast w/Exa	
☐ 53670	Catheterization Incl. Suppl	
☐ 57452	Colposcopy	
☐ 57505	ECC	
☐ 69420	Myringotomy	
☐ 92081	Visual Field Examination	
☐ 92100	Serial Tonometry Exam	
☐ 92120	Tonography	
☐ 92552	Pure Tone Audiometry	
☐ 92567	Tympanometry	
☐ 93000	Electrocardiogram	
☐ 93015	Exercise Stress Test (ETT)	
☐ 93017	ETT Tracing Only	
☐ 93040	Electrocardiogram - Rhythm	
☐ 96100	Psychological Testing	
☐ 99000	Specimen Handling	
☐ 99058	Office Emergency Care	
☐ 99070	Surgical Tray - Misc.	
☐ 99080	Special Reports of Med Rec	
☐ 99195	Phlebotomy	
☐ _____	_____	
☐ _____	_____	
☐ _____	_____	

	ICD-9 CODE DIAGNOSIS	
☐ 009.0	Ill-defined Intestinal Infect	
☐ 133.2	Establish Baseline	
☐ 174.9	Breast Cancer	
☐ 185.0	Prostate Cancer	
☐ 250	Diabetes Mellitus	
☐ 272.4	Hyperlipidemia	
☐ 282.5	Anemia - Sickle Trait	
☐ 282.60	Anemia - Sickle Cell	
☐ 285.9	Anemia, Unspecified	
☐ 300.4	Neurotic Depression	
☐ 340	Multiple Sclerosis	
☐ 342.9	Hemiplegia - Unspecified	
☐ 346.9	Migraine Headache	
☐ 352.9	Cranial Neuralgia	
☐ 354.0	Carpal Tunnel Syndrome	
☐ 355.0	Sciatic Nerve Root Lesion	
☐ 366.9	Cataract	
☐ 386.0	Vertigo	
☐ 401.1	Essential Hypertension	
☐ 414.9	Ischemic Hearth Disease	
☐ 428.0	Congestive Heart Failure	

	ICD-9 CODE DIAGNOSIS	
☐ 435.0	Basilar Artery Syndrome	
☐ 440.0	Atherosclerosis	
☐ 442.81	Carotid Artery	
☐ 460.0	Common Cold	
☐ 461.9	Acute Sinusitis	
☐ 474.0	Tonsillitis	
☐ 477.9	Hay Fever	
☐ 487.0	Flu	
☐ 496	Chronic Airway Obstruction	
☐ 522	Low Red Blood Count	
☐ 524.6	Temporo-Mandibular Jnt Synd	
☐ 538.8	Stomach Pain	
☐ 553.3	Hiatal Hernia	
☐ 564.1	Spastic Colon	
☐ 571.4	Chronic Hepatitis	
☐ 571.5	Cirrhosis of Liver	
☐ 573.3	Hepatitis	
☐ 575.2	Obstruction of Gallbladder	
☐ 648.2	Anemia - Compl. Pregnancy	
☐ 715.90	Osteoarthritis - Unspec	
☐ 721.3	Lumbar Osteo/Spondylarthrit	

	ICD-9 CODE DIAGNOSIS	
☐ 724.2	Pain: Lower Back	
☐ 727.6	Rupture of Achilles Tendon	
☐ 780.1	Hallucinations	
☐ 780.3	Convulsions	
☐ 780.5	Sleep Disturbances	
☒ 783.0	Anorexia	
☐ 783.1	Abnormal Weight Gain	
☐ 783.2	Abnormal Weight Loss	
☐ 830.6	Dislocated Hip	
☐ 830.9	Dislocated Shoulder	
☐ 841.2	Sprained Wrist	
☐ 842.5	Sprained Ankle	
☐ 891.2	Fractured Tibia	
☐ 892.0	Fractured Fibula	
☐ 919.5	Insect Bite, Nonvenomous	
☐ 921.1	Contus Eyelid/Perioc Area	
☐ v16.3	Fam. Hist of Breast Cancer	
☐ v17.4	Fam. Hist of Cardiovasc Dis	
☐ v20.2	Well Child	
☐ v22.0	Pregnancy - First Normal	
☐ v22.1	Pregnancy - Normal	

Previous Balance	Today's Charges	Total Due	Amount Paid	New Balance
_____	_____	_____	$10 check #1029	_____

Follow Up

PRN _____ Weeks _____ Months _____ Units _____

Next Appointment Date: April 30   Time: 10:30 General

Check-up

30 minutes

I hereby authorize release of any information acquired in the course of examination or treatment and allow a photocopy of my signature to be used.

_____

Figure 8-22 Encounter Form – Pamela Jermone

Sydney Carrington & Associates P.A.
34 Sycamore Street   Suite 300
Madison, CA 95653

Date: 04/16/2003

Voucher No.: 1034

Time:

Patient: Pamela Jermone
Guarantor:

Patient No: 337.0
Doctor: 1 - J. Monroe

	CPT	DESCRIPTION	FEE
	OFFICE/HOSPITAL CONSULTS		
☐	99201	Office New:Focused Hx-Exam	____
☐	99202	Office New:Expanded Hx-Exam	____
☐	99211	Office Estb:Min/None Hx-Exa	____
☐	99212	Office Estb:Focused Hx-Exam	____
☐	99213	Office Estb:Expanded Hx-Exa	____
☒	99214	Office Estb:Detailed Hx-Exa	$50
☐	99215	Office Estb:Comprhn Hx-Exam	____
☐	99221	Hosp. Initial:Comprh Hx-	____
☐	99223	Hosp.Ini:Comprh Hx-Exam/Hi	____
☐	99231	Hosp. Subsequent: S-Fwd	____
☐	99232	Hosp. Subsequent: Comprhn Hx	____
☐	99233	Hosp. Subsequent: Ex/Hi	____
☐	99238	Hospital Visit Discharge Ex	____
☐	99371	Telephone Consult - Simple	____
☐	99372	Telephone Consult - Intermed	____
☐	99373	Telephone Consult - Complex	____
☐	90843	Counseling - 25 minutes	____
☐	90844	Counseling - 50 minutes	____
☐	90865	Counseling - Special Interview	____
	IMMUNIZATIONS/INJECTIONS		
☐	90586	BCG Vaccine	____
☐	90659	Influenza Virus Vaccine	____
☐	90701	Immunization-DTP	____
☐	90702	DT Vaccine	____
☐	90703	Tetanus Toxoids	____
☐	90732	Pneumococcal Vaccine	____
☐	90746	Hepatitis B Vaccine	____
☐	90749	Immunization, Unlisted	____

	CPT	DESCRIPTION	FEE
	LABORATORY/RADIOLOGY		
☒	81000	Urinalysis	$8
☐	81002	Urinalysis; Pregnancy Test	____
☐	82951	Glucose Tolerance Test	____
☐	84478	Triglycerides	____
☐	84550	Uric Acid: Blood Chemistry	____
☐	84830	Ovulation Test	____
☐	85014	Hematocrit	____
☐	85031	Hemogram, Complete Blood Wk	____
☐	86403	Particle Agglutination Test	____
☐	86485	Skin Test; Candida	____
☐	86580	TB Intradermal Test	____
☐	86585	TB Tine Test	____
☐	87070	Culture	____
☐	70190	X-Ray, Optic Foramina	____
☐	70210	X-Ray Sinuses Complete	____
☐	71010	Radiological Exam Ent Spine	____
☐	71020	X-Ray Chest Pa & Lat	____
☐	72050	X-Ray Spine, Cerv (4 views)	____
☐	72090	X-Ray Spine; Scoliosis Ex	____
☐	72110	Spine, lumbosacral; a/p & Lat	____
☐	73030	Shoulder-Comp, min w/ 2vws	____
☐	73070	Elbow, anteropost & later vws	____
☐	73120	X-Ray; Hand, 2 views	____
☐	73560	X-Ray; Knee, 1 or 2 views	____
☐	74022	X-Ray; Abdomen, Complete	____
☐	75552	Cardiac Magnetic Res Img	____
☐	76020	X-Ray; Bone Age Studies	____
☐	76088	Mammary Ductogram Complete	____
☐	78465	Myocardial Perfusion Img	____

	CPT	DESCRIPTION	FEE
	PROCEDURES/TESTS		
☐	00452	Anesthesia for Rad Surgery	____
☐	11100	Skin Biopsy	____
☐	15852	Dressing Change	____
☐	29075	Cast Appl. - Lower Arm	____
☐	29530	Strapping of Knee	____
☐	29705	Removal/Revis of Cast w/Exa	____
☐	53670	Catheterization Incl. Suppl	____
☐	57452	Colposcopy	____
☐	57505	ECC	____
☐	69420	Myringotomy	____
☐	92081	Visual Field Examination	____
☐	92100	Serial Tonometry Exam	____
☐	92120	Tonography	____
☐	92552	Pure Tone Audiometry	____
☐	92567	Tympanometry	____
☒	93000	Electrocardiogram	$57
☐	93015	Exercise Stress Test (ETT)	____
☐	93017	ETT Tracing Only	____
☐	93040	Electrocardiogram - Rhythm	____
☐	96100	Psychological Testing	____
☐	99000	Specimen Handling	____
☐	99058	Office Emergency Care	____
☐	99070	Surgical Tray - Misc.	____
☐	99080	Special Reports of Med Rec	____
☐	99195	Phlebotomy	____
☐		_____	____
☐		_____	____
☐		_____	____

	ICD-9 CODE DIAGNOSIS	
☐	009.0	Ill-defined Intestinal Infect
☐	133.2	Establish Baseline
☐	174.9	Breast Cancer
☐	185.0	Prostate Cancer
☐	250	Diabetes Mellitus
☐	272.4	Hyperlipidemia
☐	282.5	Anemia - Sickle Trait
☐	282.60	Anemia - Sickle Cell
☐	285.9	Anemia, Unspecified
☐	300.4	Neurotic Depression
☐	340	Multiple Sclerosis
☐	342.9	Hemiplegia - Unspecified
☐	346.9	Migraine Headache
☐	352.9	Cranial Neuralgia
☐	354.0	Carpal Tunnel Syndrome
☐	355.0	Sciatic Nerve Root Lesion
☐	366.9	Cataract
☐	386.0	Vertigo
☐	401.1	Essential Hypertension
☐	414.9	Ischemic Hearth Disease
☐	428.0	Congestive Heart Failure

	ICD-9 CODE DIAGNOSIS	
☐	435.0	Basilar Artery Syndrome
☐	440.0	Atherosclerosis
☐	442.81	Carotid Artery
☐	460.0	Common Cold
☐	461.9	Acute Sinusitis
☐	474.0	Tonsillitis
☐	477.9	Hay Fever
☐	487.0	Flu
☐	496	Chronic Airway Obstruction
☐	522	Low Red Blood Count
☐	524.6	Temporo-Mandibular Jnt Synd
☐	538.8	Stomach Pain
☐	553.3	Hiatal Hernia
☐	564.1	Spastic Colon
☐	571.4	Chronic Hepatitis
☐	571.5	Cirrhosis of Liver
☐	573.3	Hepatitis
☐	575.2	Obstruction of Gallbladder
☐	648.2	Anemia - Compl. Pregnancy
☐	715.90	Osteoarthritis - Unspec
☐	721.3	Lumbar Osteo/Spondylarthrit

	ICD-9 CODE DIAGNOSIS	
☐	724.2	Pain: Lower Back
☐	727.6	Rupture of Achilles Tendon
☐	780.1	Hallucinations
☐	780.3	Convulsions
☐	780.5	Sleep Disturbances
☐	783.0	Anorexia
☐	783.1	Abnormal Weight Gain
☐	783.2	Abnormal Weight Loss
☐	830.6	Dislocated Hip
☐	830.9	Dislocated Shoulder
☐	841.2	Sprained Wrist
☐	842.5	Sprained Ankle
☐	891.2	Fractured Tibia
☐	892.0	Fractured Fibula
☐	919.5	Insect Bite, Nonvenomous
☐	921.1	Contus Eyelid/Periob Area
☐	v16.3	Fam. Hist of Breast Cancer
☐	v17.4	Fam. Hist of Cardiovasc Dis
☐	v20.2	Well Child
☐	v22.0	Pregnancy - First Normal
☐	v22.1	Pregnancy - Normal
☒	480.0	Viral Pneumonia

Previous Balance	Today's Charges	Total Due	Amount Paid	New Balance
____	____	____	$5 check #103	____

Follow Up

PRN _____ Weeks _____ Months _____ Units _____

Next Appointment Date: April 21   Time: 9:15 Recheck

I hereby authorize release of any information acquired in the course of examination or treatment and allow a photocopy of my signature to be used.

_____

_____

Figure 8-23 Encounter Form – Joseph Stewart

Sydney Carrington & Associates P.A.
34 Sycamore Street   Suite 300
Madison, CA 95653

Date: 04/16/2003

Time:

Patient: Joseph Stewart
Guarantor:

Voucher No.: 1035

Patient No: 339.0
Doctor: 3 - S. Carrington

	CPT	DESCRIPTION	FEE
	OFFICE/HOSPITAL CONSULTS		
☐	99201	Office New:Focused Hx-Exam	____
☐	99202	Office New:Expanded Hx-Exam	____
☐	99211	Office Estb:Min/None Hx-Exa	____
☐	99212	Office Estb:Focused Hx-Exam	____
☒	99213	Office Estb:Expanded Hx-Exa	$40
☐	99214	Office Estb:Detailed Hx-Exa	____
☐	99215	Office Estb:Comprhn Hx-Exam	____
☐	99221	Hosp. Initial:Comprh Hx-	____
☐	99223	Hosp.Ini:Comprh Hx-Exam/Hi	____
☐	99231	Hosp. Subsequent: S-Fwd	____
☐	99232	Hosp. Subsequent: Comprhn Hx	____
☐	99233	Hosp. Subsequent: Ex/Hi	____
☐	99238	Hospital Visit Discharge Ex	____
☐	99371	Telephone Consult - Simple	____
☐	99372	Telephone Consult - Intermed	____
☐	99373	Telephone Consult - Complex	____
☐	90843	Counseling - 25 minutes	____
☐	90844	Counseling - 50 minutes	____
☐	90865	Counseling - Special Interview	____
	IMMUNIZATIONS/INJECTIONS		
☐	90585	BCG Vaccine	____
☐	90659	Influenza Virus Vaccine	____
☐	90701	Immunization-DTP	____
☐	90702	DT Vaccine	____
☐	90703	Tetanus Toxoids	____
☐	90732	Pneumococcal Vaccine	____
☐	90746	Hepatitis B Vaccine	____
☐	90749	Immunization; Unlisted	____

	CPT	DESCRIPTION	FEE
	LABORATORY/RADIOLOGY		
☒	81000	Urinalysis	$8
☐	81002	Urinalysis; Pregnancy Test	____
☐	82951	Glucose Tolerance Test	____
☐	84478	Triglycerides	____
☐	84550	Uric Acid: Blood Chemistry	____
☐	84830	Ovulation Test	____
☐	85014	Hematocrit	____
☐	85031	Hemogram, Complete Blood Wk	____
☐	86403	Particle Agglutination Test	____
☐	86485	Skin Test; Candida	____
☐	86580	TB Intradermal Test	____
☐	86585	TB Tine Test	____
☐	87070	Culture	____
☐	70190	X-Ray; Optic Foramina	____
☐	70210	X-Ray Sinuses Complete	____
☐	71010	Radiological Exam Ent Spine	____
☐	71020	X-Ray Chest Pa & Lat	____
☐	72050	X-Ray Spine, Cerv (4 views)	____
☐	72090	X-Ray Spine; Scoliosis Ex	____
☐	72110	Spine, lumbosacral; a/p & Lat	____
☐	73030	Shoulder-Comp, min w/ 2vws	____
☐	73070	Elbow, anteropost & later vws	____
☐	73120	X-Ray; Hand, 2 views	____
☐	73560	X-Ray, Knee, 1 or 2 views	____
☐	74022	X-Ray; Abdomen, Complete	____
☐	75552	Cardiac Magnetic Res Img	____
☐	76020	X-Ray; Bone Age Studies	____
☐	76088	Mammary Ductogram Complete	____
☐	78465	Myocardial Perfusion Img	____

	CPT	DESCRIPTION	FEE
	PROCEDURES/TESTS		
☐	00452	Anesthesia for Rad Surgery	____
☐	11100	Skin Biopsy	____
☐	15852	Dressing Change	____
☐	29075	Cast Appl. - Lower Arm	____
☐	29530	Strapping of Knee	____
☐	29705	Removal/Revis of Cast w/Exa	____
☐	53670	Catheterization Incl. Suppl	____
☐	57452	Colposcopy	____
☐	57505	ECC	____
☐	69420	Myringotomy	____
☐	92081	Visual Field Examination	____
☐	92100	Serial Tonometry Exam	____
☐	92120	Tonography	____
☐	92552	Pure Tone Audiometry	____
☐	92567	Tympanometry	____
☐	93000	Electrocardiogram	____
☐	93015	Exercise Stress Test (ETT)	____
☐	93017	ETT Tracing Only	____
☐	93040	Electrocardiogram - Rhythm	____
☐	96100	Psychological Testing	____
☐	99000	Specimen Handling	____
☐	99058	Office Emergency Care	____
☐	99070	Surgical Tray - Misc.	____
☐	99080	Special Reports of Med Rec	____
☐	99195	Phlebotomy	____
☐		_____	____
☐		_____	____
☐		_____	____

	ICD-9 CODE DIAGNOSIS	
☐	009.0	Ill-defined Intestinal Infect
☐	133.2	Establish Baseline
☐	174.9	Breast Cancer
☐	185.0	Prostate Cancer
☐	250	Diabetes Mellitus
☐	272.4	Hyperlipidemia
☐	282.5	Anemia - Sickle Trait
☐	282.60	Anemia - Sickle Cell
☐	285.9	Anemia, Unspecified
☐	300.4	Neurotic Depression
☐	340	Multiple Sclerosis
☐	342.9	Hemiplegia - Unspecified
☐	346.9	Migraine Headache
☐	352.9	Cranial Neuralgia
☐	354.0	Carpal Tunnel Syndrome
☐	355.5	Sciatic Nerve Root Lesion
☐	366.9	Cataract
☐	386.0	Vertigo
☐	401.1	Essential Hypertension
☐	414.9	Ischemic Hearth Disease
☐	428.0	Congestive Heart Failure

	ICD-9 CODE DIAGNOSIS	
☐	435.0	Basilar Artery Syndrome
☐	440.0	Atherosclerosis
☐	442.81	Carotid Artery
☐	460.0	Common Cold
☐	461.9	Acute Sinusitis
☐	474.0	Tonsillitis
☐	477.9	Hay Fever
☐	487.0	Flu
☐	496	Chronic Airway Obstruction
☐	522	Low Red Blood Count
☐	524.6	Temporo-Mandibular Jnt Synd
☐	538.8	Stomach Pain
☐	553.3	Hiatal Hernia
☐	564.1	Spastic Colon
☐	571.4	Chronic Hepatitis
☐	571.5	Cirrhosis of Liver
☐	573.3	Hepatitis
☐	575.2	Obstruction of Gallbladder
☐	648.2	Anemia - Compl. Pregnancy
☐	715.90	Osteoarthritis - Unspec
☐	721.3	Lumbar Osteo/Spondylarthrit

	ICD-9 CODE DIAGNOSIS	
☒	724.2	Pain: Lower Back
☐	727.6	Rupture of Achilles Tendon
☐	780.1	Hallucinations
☐	780.3	Convulsions
☐	780.5	Sleep Disturbances
☐	783.0	Anorexia
☐	783.1	Abnormal Weight Gain
☐	783.2	Abnormal Weight Loss
☐	830.6	Dislocated Hip
☐	830.9	Dislocated Shoulder
☐	841.2	Sprained Wrist
☐	842.5	Sprained Ankle
☐	891.2	Fractured Tibia
☐	892.0	Fractured Fibula
☐	919.5	Insect Bite, Nonvenomous
☐	921.1	Contus Eyelid/Perioc Area
☐	v16.3	Fam. Hist of Breast Cancer
☐	v17.4	Fam. Hist of Cardiovasc Dis
☐	v20.2	Well Child
☐	v22.0	Pregnancy - First Normal
☐	v22.1	Pregnancy - Normal

Previous Balance	Today's Charges	Total Due	Amount Paid	New Balance
_____	_____	_____	$5 check #2003	

Follow Up

PRN _____ Weeks _____ Months _____ Units _____

Next Appointment Date: April 17 Time: 1:30 X-ray

I hereby authorize release of any information acquired in the course of
examination or treatment and allow a photocopy of my signature to be used.

EXERCISE 3: ADD A DEPENDENT TO AN EXISTING ACCOUNT

1. Use Figure 8-24 to enter a dependent to Gerald Gilmore's account.

Figure 8-24 Patient Registration – Sondra Gilmore

Patient Registration Form

Sydney Carrington & Associates
34 Sycamore Street ● Madison, CA 95653

TODAY'S DATE: _04/16/2003_

FOR OFFICE USE ONLY	
ACCOUNT NO.:	**338**
DOCTOR:	**#2**
BILL TYPE:	**11**
EXTENDED INFO.:	**0**

PATIENT INFORMATION

Gilmore   _Sondra_
PATIENT LAST NAME   FIRST NAME   MI

Wife
RELATIONSHIP TO GUARANTOR

_F_ | _06-23-54_ | _Married_ | _017-31-5416_
SEX (M/F)   DATE OF BIRTH   MARITAL STATUS   SOC. SEC. #

EMPLOYER OR SCHOOL NAME

ADDRESS OF EMPLOYER OR SCHOOL

CITY   STATE   ZIP CODE

EMPLOYER OR SCHOOL PHONE   REFERRED BY
Richard Bardsley, MD

E-MAIL

GUARANTOR INFORMATION

Gilmore   _Gerald_   _M_
RESPONSIBLE PARTY LAST NAME   FIRST NAME   MI   SEX (M/F)

89 Galley Road
MAILING ADDRESS   STREET ADDRESS (IF DIFFERENT)

Sacramento   _CA_ | _94056_
CITY   STATE   ZIP CODE

_(906) 331-2065_ | _(906) 271-9003_
(AREA CODE) HOME PHONE   (AREA CODE) WORK PHONE

_04-07-53_ | _Married_ | _132-54-7113_
DATE OF BIRTH   MARITAL STATUS   SOC. SEC. #

AutoWorks
EMPLOYER NAME

13 Bellaire Avenue
EMPLOYER ADDRESS

Sacramento   _CA_ | _94056_
CITY   STATE   ZIP CODE

PRIMARY INSURANCE

Pan American Health Ins.
NAME OF PRIMARY INSURANCE COMPANY

4567 Newberry Road
ADDRESS

Los Angeles   _CA_ | _98706_
CITY   STATE   ZIP CODE

_132-54-7113_ | _AutoWorks_
IDENTIFICATION #   GROUP NAME AND/OR #

Gerald Gilmore
INSURED PERSON'S NAME (IF DIFFERENT FROM THE RESPONSIBLE PARTY)

Same
ADDRESS (IF DIFFERENT)

Same
CITY   STATE   ZIP CODE

_(213) 456-7654_ | _132-54-7113_
PRIMARY INSURANCE PHONE NUMBER   SOC. SEC. #

Self
WHAT IS THE RESPONSIBLE PARTY'S RELATIONSHIP TO THE INSURED?

SECONDARY INSURANCE

NAME OF SECONDARY INSURANCE COMPANY

ADDRESS

CITY   STATE   ZIP CODE

IDENTIFICATION #   GROUP NAME AND/OR #

INSURED PERSON'S NAME (IF DIFFERENT FROM THE RESPONSIBLE PARTY)

ADDRESS (IF DIFFERENT)

CITY   STATE   ZIP CODE

SECONDARY INSURANCE PHONE NUMBER   SOC. SEC. #

WHAT IS THE RESPONSIBLE PARTY'S RELATIONSHIP TO THE INSURED?

I hereby consent for Sydney Carrington & Associates, P.A. to use or disclose my health information to carry out treatment, payment, and health care operations. I authorize the use of this signature on all insurance submissions. I understand that I am financially responsible for all charges whether or not paid by the insurance. I acknowledge receipt of the practice's privacy policy.

Sondra Gilmore   _04/16/2003_
PATIENT SIGNATURE   DATE

EXERCISE 4: EDIT PATIENT ACCOUNT INFORMATION

1. Based on the information provided, update patient accounts.

   a. Change Joseph Stewart's apartment number to 307 and telephone number to (906) 245-1957.

   b. For Steven Sega's work phone number add a work extension of 3996 to account.

   c. Add the group name 'Bell' to Linda Century's insurance information.

EXERCISE 5: EDIT APPOINTMENTS

1. Based on the information provided, update patient appointments.

   a. Pamela Jermone called to reschedule her recheck appointment for 11:30 on April 21.

   b. Steven Sega called to cancel his appointment.

U N I T 9

Today's
Medical Office

In the unit exercises that follow, you will print a Patient Consent report, prepare an Authorization form, and record a disclosure on a patient's account.

NOTE: The patients listed in Figures 9-1a and 91b may vary depending on exercises from previous units.

EXERCISE 1: RUN THE PRIVACY SYSTEM PATIENT CONSENT REPORT

GOAL(S): In this exercise you will print the Privacy System Patient Consent report.

1. Run the Privacy System Patient Consent report in account order for all accounts.

2. Leave the 'Only Patients Seen Since' field blank.

3. Print the report.

Figure 9-1a Patient Consent Report

```
04/16/03                    PATIENT CONSENT REPORT                    Page 1
                        Sydney Carrington & Associates P.A.
                           Account Order, All Status
                                  All Dates

Patient #        Name                        DOL Visit      Consent on File
-------------------------------------------------------------------------------
   300.1         Walters Theresa L                               Yes
   301.1         Carlos Helena                                   Yes
   302.0         Glenmore Edward R                               Yes
   303.1         Monaco Nancy                                    NO
   304.0         Monti Vincent A                                 Yes
   305.0         Viajo Catherine A           04/16/2003          Yes
   305.1         Viajo Michael                                   Yes
   306.0         Cusack Christine G          04/16/2003          Yes
   306.1         Cusack Richard                                  Yes
   307.0         Wyatt John                  04/16/2003          Yes
   308.0         Frost William               04/16/2003          Yes
   308.1         Frost Linda                 04/16/2003          Yes
   309.0         Perez Juan                  04/16/2003          Yes
   310.0         Cruz Rebecca                04/16/2003          Yes
   310.1         Noonan Matthew              04/16/2003          Yes
   311.0         Vega Roberto R              04/16/2003          Yes
   312.0         Salvani William                                 Yes
   312.1         Salvani Christopher                             Yes
   312.2         Salvani Kyle M                                  Yes
   313.0         Stein Erin R                                    Yes
   314.0         Fuentas Carmen P                                Yes
   314.1         Fuentas David                                   Yes
   315.0         Morgan Margaret F           01/10/2003          Yes
   315.1         Morgan Brian                                    Yes
   315.2         Morgan Peter                                    Yes
   316.0         Barker Sharon               01/10/2003          Yes
   316.1         Barker Richard                                  Yes
   316.2         Barker Sarah                                    Yes
   317.0         Lopez Sonia A               04/16/2003          Yes
   318.0         Brinkman Gary               04/17/2003          Yes
   319.0         Miles Wayne P               04/16/2003          Yes
   319.1         Miles Sheila                                    Yes
   320.0         Ramirez Leanna M            04/16/2003          Yes
   321.0         Marchese Anna S             04/16/2003          Yes
   321.1         Marchese Nicholas                               Yes
   322.0         Santos Paul R               04/16/2003          Yes
   322.1         Santos Carol                04/16/2003          Yes
   323.0         Weiland Candace             04/16/2003          Yes
   323.1         Weiland Stephen             04/16/2003          Yes
   324.0         Hatcher Craig M             01/10/2003          Yes
   325.0         Roberts Ashleigh K          01/10/2003          Yes
   325.1         Roberts Renee                                   Yes
   326.0         Scheller Denise L           02/01/2003          Yes
   327.0         Fitzpatrick Mark P          02/01/2003          Yes
   327.1         Fitzpatrick Roberta                             Yes
   328.0         Penny Robert                02/15/2003          Yes
   329.0         Knifert John                02/15/2003          Yes
   330.0         Zapola Karen L              02/15/2003          Yes
   331.0         Jones Elizabeth             02/15/2003          Yes
   332.0         Walker Ross M                                   Yes
   332.1         Walker Jacqueline                               Yes
   333.0         Swindel Alan P                                  Yes
   333.1         Swindel Margaret                                Yes
```

Figure 9-1b Patient Consent Report (continued)

```
04/16/03                    PATIENT CONSENT REPORT                  Page 2
                       Sydney Carrington & Associates P.A.
                          Account Order, All Status
                                All Dates

  Patient #          Name                    DOL Visit    Consent on File
  ---------------------------------------------------------------------------
     333.2      Swindel Daniel                                 NO
     334.0      Berntson Allison                               Yes
     335.0      Cantorelli Brittany R                          Yes
     335.1      Rutger Donna                                   NO
     336.0      Valentine Michael M                            Yes
     337.0      Jermone Pamela R            04/16/2003          Yes
     338.0      Gilmore Gerald              04/16/2003          Yes
     338.1      Gilmore Sondra                                 Yes
     339.0      Stewart Joseph M            04/16/2003          Yes
     340.0      Sega Steven T               04/16/2003          Yes
     341.0      Century Linda               04/16/2003          Yes


                        Total Unknown :        0
                        Total No      :        3
                        Total Revoked :        0
                        Total Yes     :       61
```

EXERCISE 2: PREPARE AN AUTHORIZATION FORM FOR A PATIENT

GOAL(S): In this exercise you will print an Authorization form for Daniel Swindel's wrestling coach.

Daniel Swindel needs an authorization form to be completed for his wrestling coach. In order to join the wrestling team, a sports physical is required for all students. Based on the following information, prepare an Authorization form for Daniel Swindel.

1. Retrieve Daniel Swindel's account from the Patient Privacy Records screen.

2. The form will be signed by Daniel's mother.

3. The Purpose of Disclosure is a sports physical.

4. Leave Contact Party blank and complete the following fields:

   a. Authorized Party: Fairview Junior High School

   b. Attention: Wrestling Coach

   c. Address: 420 Hunter Avenue

   d. City: Madison

   e. State: CA

   f. Zip Code: 95653

5. The results of the sports physical is the information to be disclosed.

6. Compare your screen to Figure 9-2. Print the form. Compare your form to Figure 9-3.

Figure 9-2 Patient Privacy Authorization

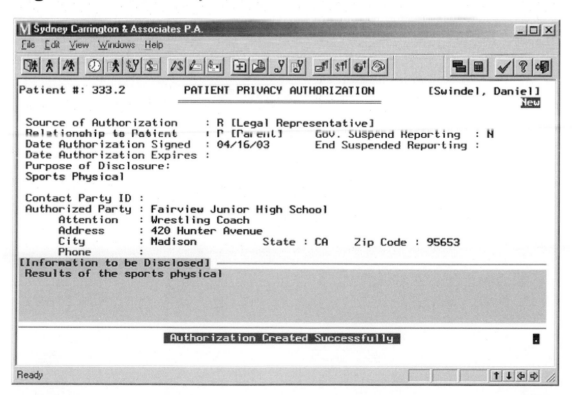

Figure 9-3 Authorization to Disclose Patient Records

AUTHORIZATION TO DISCLOSE PATIENT RECORDS

I hereby authorize Sydney Carrington & Associates P.A. to disclose individually identifiable protected health information concerning the patient:

Daniel Swindel
14 Bonekak Lane
Sacramento CA 94056

To: Wrestling Coach
     420 Hunter Avenue
     Madison, CA 95653

For the purpose of:
Sports Physical

Information to be Disclosed:
Results of the sports physical

This Authorization is to remain in effect from 04/16/2003

I understand that I have the right to revoke this authorization by notifying the practice in writing until such time as a disclosure has been made based on this authorization. In addition, I understand that my signing this authorization is not required for the practice to provide me with health care service, except if the sole purpose of the service is for the practice to provide health care information to the authorized party named in this document. Finally, I understand that the information disclosed pursuant to this authorization may be redisclosed by the authorized party and no longer be protected by the laws under which this authorization was created.

Signed _____   Date _____

Relation to Patient: Parent

EXERCISE 3: RECORD A DISCLOSURE FOR A PATIENT

GOAL(S): In this exercise you will record a disclosure for Daniel Swindel.

The results from Daniel's sports physical have been received. Based on the following information, prepare a record of disclosure, indicating that you have sent the results to his wrestling coach.

1. Retrieve Daniel Swindel's account from the Patient Privacy Records screen.

2. Select the sports physical and choose (D)isclosures.

3. Add a new disclosure record using the following information:

   a. Accept the default date for date of disclosure.

   b. Accept the default to disclose to the Authorized Party.

   c. Accept the default for the sports physical information to be disclosed.

4. Process the information. Compare your screen to Figure 9-4.

Figure 9-4 Disclosure Record

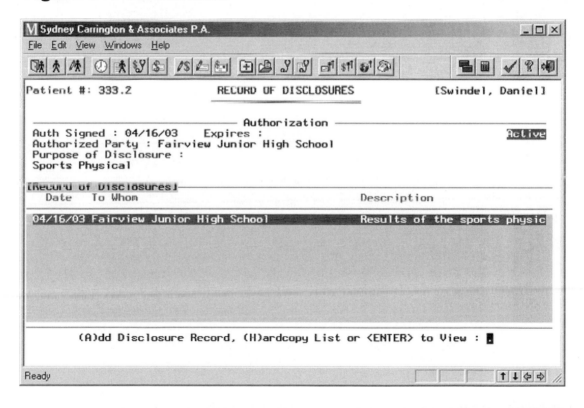